YOGA
YEARS

YOGA YEARS

True stories of how
yoga transforms ageing

KATHY ARTHURSON

Yoga Years. True stories of how yoga transforms ageing

First published in Australia 2020 by Kathy Arthurson.

Copyright © 2020 Kathy Arthurson

The moral rights of the author have been asserted.

Cover design & internal design by Zena Shapter.
Yoga position illustrations by Chathuri Sugandhika.

ISBN 978-0-6486802-4-6

A new day for you and for me.
You construct a day from the early morning light and birdsong.
I leap into the light... (Barb St John).

CONTENTS

INTRODUCTION

The number of people aged over 60 is doubling (to reach 2 billion by 2050).[1] In writing this book my aim is to draw on the knowledge and wisdom of ordinary people in this age group. I want to share how they are making sense of their lives, living life to the fullest – and refusing to descend into so-called 'old age'. When I recently celebrated my 60th birthday, I felt blessed to have reached this special milestone. My enthusiasm was soon dampened when a well-meaning (somewhat younger) acquaintance advised me to look after myself, 'because it will all be downhill from now on!'

Over time, I've become increasingly aware of the multitude of negative attitudes about growing older. Far from being harmless, identifying with these mindsets can lead to nasty consequences for our wellbeing, including increased risks of depression and social isolation.[2] It seems I'm not alone in feeling fed up with hearing stories about the *burden of ageing*; many others of my generation (and beyond) also agree that a shift in attitudes towards ageing is long overdue.[3]

For a long time now (over 20 years), I've been fascinated by older yoga teachers – their ease of movement, joy, vigour and enthusiasm for life – and they always appear a lot younger than they really are. I wondered what these teachers, with their imbued wisdom and experience, could tell us about this special time of life.

Maybe you're like me, in the second half of your life and open to hearing fresh, positive stories about ageing – stories that honour and preserve the unique wisdom and knowledge of our elders for current and future generations. Or are you perhaps just curious about the benefits of yoga and have always wanted to try it out for yourself? Possibly (like many people) you are put off by glossy images of lithe, Lycra-clad bodies bending and stretching in impossible poses! Or simply anxious that you're not flexible, athletic or young enough. Perchance you have no desire to touch your toes, but you want to read about how to live a healthy, productive life with a sense of inner contentment as you age, through making specific lifestyle choices.

Whatever your level of interest, the nine yoga teachers in this collection will help to dispel your doubts and enliven your knowledge about yoga and thriving into older age. The youngest teacher is 66, the oldest 95, and they all still practise yoga – collectively they have over 400 years of wisdom to share. These women will take you on their own humorous and heartfelt, intimate journeys with yoga and offer answers to the many questions you might have, including:

- What is the best approach to live and enjoy life as you age?
- How can yoga help you to navigate the rocky episodes of life?
- How do you find the right teacher?

- What type of yoga should you practise?
- Is yoga a cure for chronic health conditions?
- How is yoga different from a gym workout or fitness class?

In this book, you'll also read about the challenges these teachers have faced in life (just like us): when their relationships broke down or they suffered from ill health or other crises. But their individual stories show how yoga has helped each of these teachers pick up the pieces, overcome obstacles and move forward in life. Bette Calman (aged 91) and Vivien Vieritz (95) have sustained their yoga practices over more than six decades, while many of the others started yoga later in life.

The teachers here will also help you to understand that there are no limitations to practising yoga: you don't have be young or fit, or do poses that hurt or injure you. You don't have to practise difficult breathing techniques that make you dizzy, or sit uncomfortably in meditation postures.

This book offers a fresh perspective on ageing: while none of the teachers here deny that ageing is inevitable, the yoga practices they advocate will provide physical and mental benefits, as well as pathways to places of rest and stillness and inner knowing – thereby shifting ingrained attitudes about ageing. Adopting a yoga practice can help you to find a deeper meaning in life, to cope with everyday challenges with greater wisdom, and to make ageing a process of more – not less – enjoyment.

My own story about yoga

My first yoga teacher Bette Calman, who features in this book, was already in her 70s (and vibrant and strong) when I started her classes. Unlike Bette, who started yoga aged 26, my journey started later in life. While I tagged along with friends to several yoga classes in my teens, back then it seemed far too gentle a practice, and to be honest I found yoga boring. Looking back, I guess that the time just wasn't right for me and I hadn't yet found the right teacher or yoga tradition.

So, for many years I avoided yoga. However, things changed when I started a PhD in 1998: my mind was a whirlpool of endless anxiety provoking inner chatter that I simply couldn't switch off. Like many others in western society who were also struggling with stress, I turned to yoga as a therapy. I found the best part of the yoga class for me was the guided relaxation at the end: this provided a much-needed rest for the mind, a calm space at last, where anxieties about my PhD quietened and my stress dissolved. Now I was truly hooked on yoga and my life hummed along. I also finished the PhD.

In 2007, I decided to take my regular yoga practice one step further and undertake teacher training. I noticed that several teachers at the yoga classes I attended in Melbourne wore little gold badges with the word 'Gita' printed on them. Intrigued I asked the teacher after class one day, 'What's the Gita badge about?'

'Oh, Gita is just a studio down at Abbotsford where some of us trained,' was the casual reply.

I contacted the Gita studio and everything about it felt warm and inviting, from the webpage to the woman who answered my initial phone enquiry. 'Teacher training only happens every two years,' she said, 'and the next course starts this coming weekend. If you're interested, you'll need to first attend an interview with the directors of Gita: Di Lucas and Lucille Wood.'

Off I went the next day to a yoga studio I knew very little about, and sat on the other side of a desk from my interviewers, Di and Lucille, for over an hour. They asked lots of questions: Why did I want to be a yoga teacher? What would I give back to the yoga community? I answered as openly and honestly as I could.

After the interview, I was given the welcome news that I'd been accepted into the course. Lucille clicked her fingers and said, 'Coco Chanel'. Flabbergasted, I wondered what on earth Gita Yoga had to do with perfume or fashion! From under the desk emerged two black poodles: these beautiful 'Gita girls' were called Coco and Channelle. They weren't guide or companion dogs, and unbeknown to me had sat under the desk the whole time! And now, looking back on that time studying at Gita, I recall that Coco and Channelle attended all the yoga classes Lucille taught – they sat behind her, always calm and contented, at the back of the podium.

Thus I took the next step in my yoga journey that weekend to become a yoga teacher. Over the years I've continued teaching yoga classes once or twice a week in between my busy work schedule as a university researcher. My own practice has deepened and become much more than just a release from stress – it's become a way of life, a framework for ethical living, health and happiness, and discovering a community of like-minded people. On a deeper level, it's helped me to connect to the core of my being.

Now that I'm older I find that yoga is important to how I feel about ageing – and there is a growing body of evidence suggesting that yoga is beneficial for healthy ageing.[4] My curiosity ignited, I wondered what might we learn from the wisdom of seasoned yoga teachers who have travelled further down this pathway of learning about yoga and its effects on health and ageing. It may have just remained a nagging quest because there were always so many reasons to put off this research project: there was never enough time and I was too busy with other work.

The 'hurry up' call came when a dear friend, Barb St John, was diagnosed with terminal cancer. I made the decision to begin the research project in 2017. I searched the internet for yoga teachers aged 60 plus to interview, and others were suggested through my yoga networks. Before interviewing these teachers, I attended one of their classes (if they were still teaching) and found it a lovely way to connect, especially if we weren't acquainted beforehand. All the interviews were recorded and later transcribed; the selected transcriptions for this book were sent to each contributor for checking and revision rounds before their final approval. In the creation of this book, we have all been co-researchers and taken this very special yoga journey together to gather and preserve precious wisdom for future and current generations.

I learnt a great deal from the wisdom of these women that surprised and delighted me, and a lot more about vibrant ageing and yoga itself through researching this book. I've thoroughly enjoyed the journey and am thrilled to share it with you. The yoga teachers in this book continue to inspire me and I hope that as you read their personal stories about the many benefits of yoga, and of their own lives – lived well – that you will also be inspired.

#1
TANIA DYETT

KEEPING THE BODY IN GOOD HEALTH WITH YOGA

Ageing can creep up if you are unaware
~ practise yoga to delay the hardening of the body

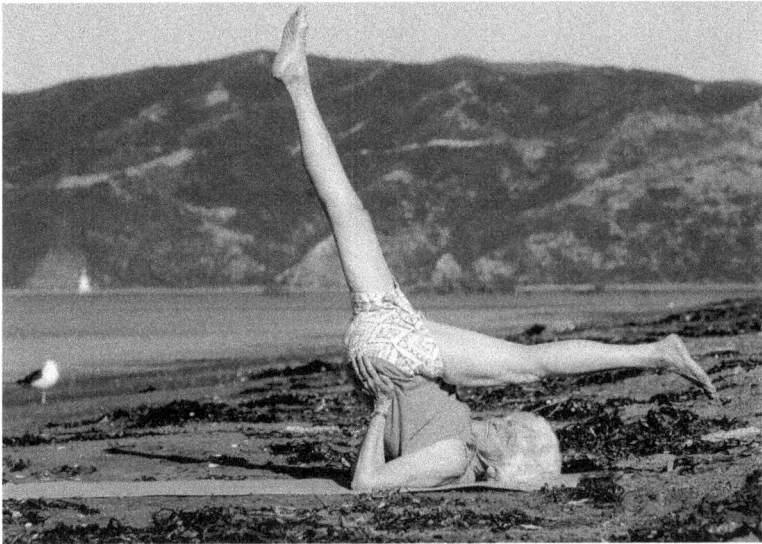

Tania practising yoga on the beach at Seatoun, New Zealand
(Stuff/Dominion Post)

Tania
Teaches us
The pussycat pose.
'Wag those tails,' she instructs.
We transform to dog pose.
Laughter then
Stillness.

Seatoun, in New Zealand, is best known for its fabulous scenery, as featured in the Lord of the Rings film trilogy. It's also the long-time home to 92-year-old Tania Dyett, who teaches one yoga class a week in St Georges Hall, a short walk from her home.

To get a taste of Tania's teaching style, I attended her Tuesday night class (which ran for 90 minutes). We flowed from one yoga pose into the next and were pampered with a delicious relaxation at the end. During class, Tania also read an inspirational poem and taught us her favourite pose, which she calls 'my pussy cat'. She started us in the cat pose then built on it, segueing from cat to dog pose, through instructing us to wag our tails! It was fun and brought a smile to my face. Tania later told me, 'Initially, when I demonstrate this sequence in class students think it's very unusual. The first time I performed it at a yoga conference the audience laughed like hell! But it's a good yoga pose to teach because it puts an image into people's minds of which part of the body they're going to work.'

I was amazed at how Tania moved down on to, and up from, the floor with ease. It was a testament to her motto that: 'Keeping your body in good health is a duty.' However, she remains quite humble about this and explained: 'The only way I can get up from the floor is by going into downward dog then moving upwards from there.'

Tania has led an inspirational life in many ways and, in her own words, has been 'a citizen of the world.' The following is Tania's tale of how, in her twenties, she attended her first yoga class in New Zealand. Along the way, routine life events diverted her from the yogic path (as they inevitably do) until eventually, aged in her fifties, she became a yoga teacher. Fast forward to today, when Tania is still teaching yoga at the spritely age of 92.

TANIA'S STORY

My early years

My father was an officer in the Russian Tsarist Army, and an assistant of Admiral Alexander Kolchak (a leader of the White Movement, who fought the Bolsheviks in the early 20th century). When Kolchak was executed by the Bolsheviks in 1920, my parents fled Russia in fear for their lives. They travelled on the Trans-Siberian Railway and managed to reach the northern part of China. There the Latvian Consul provided them with a horse each so they could travel deeper into China. They finally reached Hankau, where I was born and spent the first four and a half years of my life.

After Hankau, my family moved to the Dutch East Indies (as Indonesia was formerly known). It was there that my budding passion for playing and teaching the violin was nurtured; this was long before I discovered yoga. I remember the local mayor asking me whether I would prefer a holiday or a violin. I opted for the violin and it was actually a very good one – a copy of a Maggini.[5] Unfortunately, some time later I accidentally put my foot through this violin and it was never mended. Just as well it was an imitation and not an authentic Maggini!

During the Second World War, Japan invaded the Dutch East Indies, and my mother and I were interned in a Japanese camp in West Java. My father was sent to a separate male-only camp. At that time, I was 16 and our internment lasted for three and a half years, until the war ended and we were finally freed. Once my mother and father reunited, they wanted to migrate to Australia, however my mother had contracted tuberculosis and was deemed ineligible for entry.

Fortunately, the New Zealand government accepted us and we moved to New Zealand in 1946, soon after the Second World War had ended. I settled into life there and found office work for various organisations in New Zealand, including Red Cross and Dominion Life Insurance Company.

I have a humorous story from those days to share with you. When I was secretary for one of the managers at the life insurance company in Wellington, I had my own little office. One day there was a conference on and all the branch managers were attending. The intercom system in my office announced: 'Mrs Dyett, please come to the conference to take dictation.' Now, at the time I was still learning English and trying to speak using grammar precisely – just like in the dictionary. So, I replied through the intercom: 'I am having an intercourse with the branch manager from Auckland. I'll be there in a minute.' Well, the branch manager's face turned bright red and he dashed out of my office in a big hurry! Of course, the problem was that the dictionary definition of 'intercourse' includes an 'official conversation' and I had taken this meaning literally.

Discovering yoga and becoming a teacher

In my twenties, before my two children were born, I went along to my first yoga class, which was taught by a husband and wife team: he would guide us through the poses and explain the benefits of practising yoga, and she would demonstrate the poses for us to follow.

After some time of attending classes, one of my yoga teachers noted my flexibility and passion for yoga, and advised me to think seriously about becoming a yoga teacher. By this time, there was a yoga teacher training course running in New Zealand. Previously people had to travel to Australia for their training.

Through the International Yoga Teachers Association (IYTA), I joined Eric Doornekamp (the first local yoga teacher in New Zealand to run a teacher training course). There were only six students and the course ran for a year. I found it an excellent course, especially the invaluable grounding we were given in breathing practices. In fact, during my studies I was required to write an assignment on a specific topic of interest, and I chose to write mine on the importance of breathing properly.

Although I didn't start teaching yoga until much later in life – after raising my two children – I've actually ended up teaching for over 40 years. At one stage I only had four pupils and it looked like reducing to three. I thought, *oh, I'd better finish up with teaching,* but I'm glad I decided to continue, because now I have ten regular students, some of whom have been coming to my classes for 30 years.

Yoga means 'union' as it connects all three parts of our

existence – body, mind and spirit – so they work together in harmony. The spiritual aspect of life is often sadly neglected in this busy material world. When I teach, I illustrate different ideas by drawing on Buddhist psychology and using positive affirmations. For example: if you believe that you're sad, and you keep thinking about being sad, and telling yourself you're sad – then what happens? Not surprisingly you can't help but feel *really, really* sad. So, as much as possible, we need to counteract negative ways of thinking in life. As the Buddha once said: '*Your mind is the entity that makes it possible to be who you are*'. We make our worlds with our minds, and with our thoughts we create our minds. So, we need to keep our thoughts strong and clear; we need to stay positive, and I believe yoga helps because it can effectively moderate negative self-talk.

Ageing and injury: how yoga can help

Keeping up physical movement definitely helps with the ageing process. Over my lifetime, yoga has given me a healthy body and mind – as well as boundless energy.

Ageing doesn't just happen abruptly – it creeps up slowly if you're not aware. One day you might notice that your body feels tight in certain areas, and it's important to be aware of this tightness, as it gradually prevents or blocks the flow of *prana* (essential life force energy). I personally believe that yoga delays the hardening of the body – including its muscles, sinews, nerves and glands – through improving flexibility and strength. The *asanas* (postures) work on the endocrine system, balancing the hormones; while the body itself maintains or regains suppleness, restoring movement and releasing the internal conflicts that can harm health.

Over the years, my practice and teaching has changed in response to the circumstances of my life. In the past I could balance on one leg, but at the moment my sense of balance is limited due to a fall. I was in a hurry and tripped on the steps at the front of my house. As a result, I injured my hip and ended up in hospital, where a pin was inserted to repair the fracture. Since then, I've had another fall, but having that piece of titanium in my hip certainly helped prevent further injury! The doctors told me that the pin has made my hip stronger than it's ever been. However, I do take care these days; I don't go bike-riding any more as I'm frightened of losing my balance.

Following my hip injury, I continued to practise yoga – it helped me to recuperate quickly, and to accept what happened and move on. There are lots of postures I can't do now, especially strong ones like the handstand or headstand; but I can still manage the shoulder stand. To help with balancing poses, I place a chair in front of me for support.

It's important as you grow older to avoid certain conditions: for example, developing a dowager's hump (kyphosis) with an abnormal outward curvature of the spine and shoulders ending up around your ears. Yoga helps us to avoid this through preserving the health of the spine. In fact, I always do the reverse prayer pose because it helps my shoulders to move down, as follows:

Reverse prayer pose

(to preserve flexibility in the spine, shoulders and wrists):

- Start by relaxing into the shoulders.
- Then take your hands behind your back, fingers facing down to start, and press the fingertips together.
- Then turn the hands upwards, and try to bring the palms together so that the little fingers press into the upper back.

This is a good pose for the wrists as well; I find it assists me with playing the violin. And the body is like a musical instrument – you need to play it to keep it in good health.

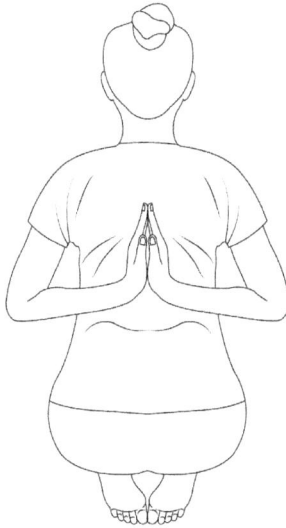

Following your passions in life

If I hadn't found yoga, I think my life would be exceedingly empty – although music has also given me lots of fun and joy. When I was younger, I performed music recitals in schools throughout New Zealand and saw many beautiful parts of the country, stretching from the North to the South Islands. In the 1980s, I did a television program about music for young people; the series was called *Time for Music* and each episode ran for about 10 minutes. I was only 59 at that time but called myself the 'old lady'. Now I'm 92! In one episode of that TV show I wanted to play some Russian music but the producer wasn't too keen, so I simply told him I didn't want to do the program anymore. The next day, a bouquet of flowers arrived with a card from the producer saying, '*You won – do your Russian program.*'

I also formed a light music string quartet and we played at weddings and social functions – even at Government House. In fact, over the years, I played for three of New Zealand's Prime Ministers, including David Lange (who was a wonderful orator, by the way).

I'm currently involved in Yoga Aotearoa, the International Yoga Teachers Association (IYTA) of New Zealand, and for a while I was on their management committee. Personally, I don't believe in committees but at the same time I do realise they're necessary to get things done.

Yoga Aotearoa held a wonderful convention in Wellington, in January 2017. I asked Lilias Folan[6] if she would present at it. Initially, she said she'd be delighted to take part in the convention but, unfortunately, found she couldn't attend, due to problems with her husband's health. I was terribly disappointed; although I've never actually met Lilias in person, she's been a major influence on my own yoga teaching style. In fact, when I first contacted Lilias about the convention, I confided that her very first book on yoga was my inspiration – my yoga bible![7]

What I love about Lilias' teaching style is that she's brilliant at explaining cues and images to give to students. For example, the way Lilias describes how to do a three-part yogic breath, is crystal clear: *'Put your thumb on the tummy button and then with the in-breath expand your ribs and feel your collarbones.'* The eye exercises she teaches are also important because the eyes are muscles too. Unfortunately, few yoga teachers include eye movements in their classes these days, but I feel they're an essential group of practices, as most people stare at computer and television screens for hours on end, fatiguing some eye muscles and not moving others. Just like other muscles in the body the eyes can benefit from a varied 'workout'.

Neither of my children practise yoga, but I believe it's more important to follow your individual passions in life. My daughter enjoys studying languages (as I do) and she's also a teacher. My son went into classical music, completing his Master of Music at Victoria University. I'm extremely proud of both my children's achievements.

My mother never did any exercises at all and she lived to the ripe old age of 92. That's the age I am now, but I'm not going yet! Yes, I'm an old lady but I intend to do yoga for the rest of my life – for the sake of my body, mind and spirit.

As the Buddha once said:

'To keep the body in good health is a duty. For otherwise we shall not be able to trim the lamp of wisdom and keep our minds strong and clear. Water surrounds the lotus flower but does not touch the petals.'[8]

REFLECTIONS

The day after I attended Tania's yoga class, we met at her home to do the interview. Tania's house is perched on a hillside engulfed with treetops and it felt like we were sitting in a forest – the views were magnificent. After the interview, we had a lovely morning tea with her son Kim and talked about all sorts of topics beyond yoga, including how Tania ended up living in her home at Seatoun. Originally Tania's parents didn't have enough money for a deposit on the property; they were assisted in purchasing it through the kindness of a retired school teacher whose brother (like Tania's family) had been detained in a Japanese prisoner of war camp in the East Indies. Sadly, he had died there.

I also heard a little more about Tania's family's roots in Russia. She told me that her parents never talked about their experiences in Russia because they must have been horrifying. What Tania does know is that her mother attended a prestigious school established by Catherine the Great, which was mainly for girls of noble birth. While Tania's mother did not belong to the nobility, her father oversaw five factories in the Urals, so the family was wealthy. This was the region where weapons manufacturing was concentrated before the collapse of the Soviet Union in 1991.

When Tania visited Moscow for the very first time in 1976, to study music teaching methods, unsurprisingly she was not permitted to visit the Urals.

Food and feijoas

Tania confided to me that she's not a vegetarian and added, 'While I do eat a lot of vegetables, I also eat fish and eggs – but not red meat or dairy.' She mentioned that sometimes to be polite she has eaten red meat that was offered to her. Displaying a touching compassion for other people's feelings, she added, 'You can't just say to people: I don't eat this or I don't eat that, especially if you are visiting someone's house and haven't sorted out your dietary requirements with them beforehand.'

Tania and Kim also introduced me to a New Zealand favourite, the feijoa. I had to confess that I'd never tasted one before. For those who aren't familiar with feijoas, they're an egg-shaped fruit with a lime-green skin. To me, the jelly-like centre tasted a bit like a mixture of strawberries, pineapples and guava – very unusual but quite refreshing. As I departed, Tania gave me a big bag of feijoas to take with me. We strolled down the road together towards the Seatoun Esplanade, enjoying the stunning 'Lord of the Rings' type scenery. Along the way Tania left me to walk alone as she dropped in to visit a friend.

What I learnt from Tania (in a nutshell)

I meandered back to my accommodation, mulling over Tania's

viewpoint about negative mindsets placing limits on our health and wellbeing – and how practising yoga frees our minds, opening us up to new possibilities. I also reflected on her idea about 'ageing with awareness' – as she emphasised that ageing creeps up if you're unaware. Tania is a perfect example of what she advocates: keeping physically active through sustaining her yoga practice, making conscious decisions about how to live well, staying connected with her students and still learning, giving and having a purpose in life.

People like Tania make our world a much better place.

#2
MAGGIE COOMBS

YOGA IS THE BEST OPTION

Learn to accept the unchangeable with grace and serenity
and to transform rocky moments into periods of growth

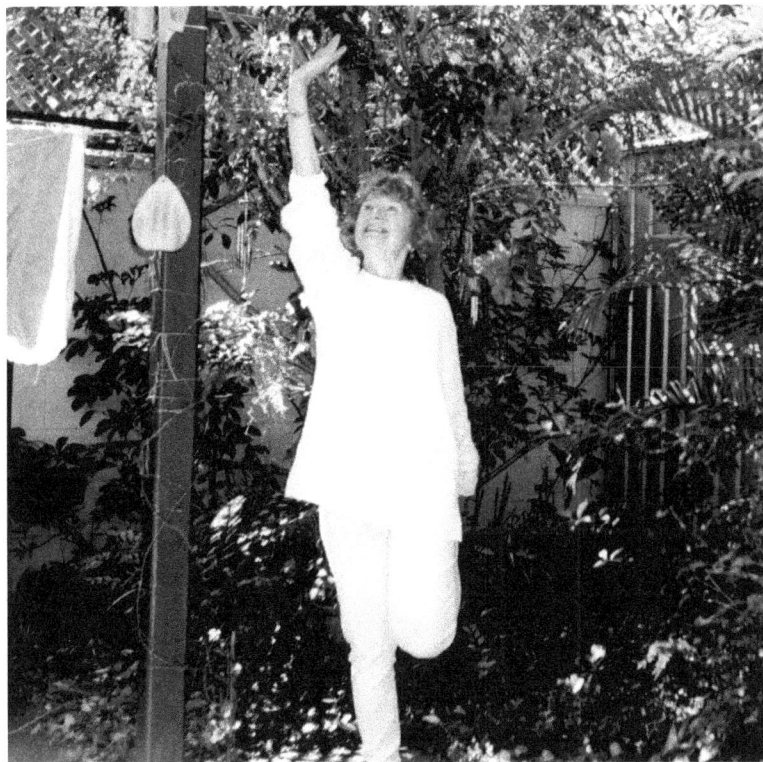

Maggie practising yoga in her garden

Maggie
At eighty
Resides on Bribie
Teaching yoga therapy
Under the gum trees.
Precious gift
For all!

Maggie lives on beautiful Bribie Island, on Queensland's Sunshine Coast. When I arrived to participate in her Tuesday morning yoga class, she immediately struck me as a warm, vibrant person with radiant red hair and sparkling eyes; she also greeted me with a hug! I was touched by her peaceful presence throughout the class – sentiments that were later reinforced when we met to do our interview.

Maggie's class was remedial yoga and relaxation, starting outside with pranayama (breathing practices) under the gum trees; tuning into the breath we were bathed in warm dappled sunlight. Then we moved into the church hall for the remainder of the class, which included plenty of gentle limbering and stretching exercises, followed by a series of balancing and classical asanas, which were slow-paced and practised with awareness of how our bodies were feeling. All this was wonderfully calming.

As Maggie was recovering from a recent hip replacement operation, she couldn't demonstrate all the poses. Instead, she taught off the mat (like several of the other yoga teachers featured in this book), bearing testament to one of the many invaluable skills honed over almost 50 continuous years of teaching. Maggie's style of teaching included calling out the name of each pose, describing with precision how to move into and out of it, then assisting her students where appropriate.

After the class had finished, I headed off alone to a local café to prepare for our interview, giving Maggie time to pack up and say goodbye to her students. As I was leaving the hall, one of Maggie's students asked me how I found the class. When I told her how peaceful I felt, she nodded and replied: 'Every time

I come to Maggie's class, I feel so calm and relaxed – and the feeling of peace lasts all day.'

When we started the interview, Maggie noted that there had been 16 students that day in the class, which was a little larger than usual. Revealing a delightful and quirky sense of humour, she confided: 'Well, to make a living as a yoga teacher you need enough students to put some butter on your bread.'

The following is Maggie's story of her travels with her yoga mat, and how she came to be teaching therapeutic yoga at the age of 80 on Bribie Island.

MAGGIE'S STORY

Finding yoga and becoming a teacher

I discovered yoga in the late 1960s, when I was living in Sydney and my marriage was breaking down. I needed to find strength and coping mechanisms, and I certainly didn't want to turn to alcohol or 'bad' men. My sister suggested that I try yoga, so I started classes with Nicolas Volin, Michael Volin's twin brother.[9] When I first met Nicolas, he was teaching in different venues around Sydney, including Manly and the northern suburbs. I used to follow his timetable, going from place to place to attend two or three of his classes each week. I received so much benefit from yoga – it was during the time before I finally left my husband and was stressed beyond belief.

Thoughts turned to becoming a teacher myself, and one day I very cheekily told Nicolas that I wanted to teach yoga. He was open to the idea, advising me that I was quite good at most of the poses, except for the shoulder stand.

So, in order to become a yoga teacher I had to master the shoulder stand. Nicolas was confident that I could conduct a class, because prior to taking up yoga I was already a dance instructor. He started to train me in the 'traditional' way: one-on-one, teacher-to-student instruction. As I was the only student that made the training feel extra special. During my training I was required to explain and then demonstrate each of the yoga postures, and at the end of the session I would give a guided relaxation practice. However, I found the training very slow. In 1971, I did one of Swami Sarasvati's[10] classes, and ended up joining her yoga teacher training course, while still being trained by Nicolas. After completing Swami Sarasvati's teacher training, I felt compelled to confess to Nicolas what had happened, and that I was now a qualified yoga teacher. All he said was, 'Oh, well you'd better teach some of my classes then.'

It was an extraordinary time for me because I was teaching classes for some of the people who first introduced yoga in Australia. Nicolas would also ask me to take Nancy Phelan's classes when she went away. Nancy Phelan[11] was wonderful; I still have some of the marvellous books she wrote about yoga with Michael Volin. Nancy would travel around the city on buses and write notes for her books on the bus tickets! Although, to be absolutely correct, this group of people were not quite the first to teach yoga in Australia; there was a generation before them, mainly men who were based in Sydney. One of these, Russell Frank Atkinson, started teaching Hatha Yoga in the late 1940s in Sydney. He also published numerous books and gave me a copy of his hilarious *Diary of a Dropout* (Wellspring 1990).[12]

Another yogi who greatly influenced my teaching was Acharya (Upendra Chandra Roy)[13], although he didn't really start teaching yoga in Australia until the late 1960s. I attended his yoga teacher training course twice weekly; the classes were conducted in a lofty studio in an old building in Day Street, Sydney (where he also lived). Acharya used Sanskrit names for the yoga poses and would shift from one posture to the next, and his students would move through each posture with him. That was his way of teaching and I also adopted elements of his teaching style for my own classes.

Looking back to those early days of Australian yoga, it was taught in the 'traditional' way: as a complete system incorporating *asanas*, yoga philosophy and spiritual teachings. There are so many variants of traditional yoga now, and other disciplines mixed with yoga. In my view it's become 'watered-down' yoga: fashionable and trendy. Teachers are popping up all over the place who do quick courses and gain certification without much depth of traditional knowledge.

Discovering the Yoga for Health Foundation

After teaching for some time, I injured my back in a car accident. Fortunately, I didn't break any bones but there was extensive soft tissue damage. The pain was unbearable and I could hardly stand or walk. I tried to find a yoga class to attend that didn't aggravate my back, as strong classes were no good at all.

In the 1970s, I came across the Yoga for Health Foundation,

which had been founded in the UK by a man called Howard Kent (who was also the director). In 1971, there was even a UK-based *Yoga for Health* TV series and the Foundation began to extend its activities to other countries, including Australia. The appeal for me was that these people taught sensitively, with a special focus on breath awareness, and using gentle *pranayama* to improve the breath and bring it to its optimum natural state. These teachers also modified the postures for different bodies and health conditions, and usually had smaller class sizes. I loved this style of yoga from the moment I tried it; in fact, I was so enthralled with their therapeutic way of teaching that I joined a weekend training in Sydney with Sophia Brandjes (the one-time president of *Yoga for Health* in Australia).

Yoga for Health also had a mentoring system, and used the one-on-one teaching style of traditional yoga, which was so deeply beneficial and supportive for me. I had a friend who taught nearby at that time; we both belonged to the committee for *Yoga for Health* and spent hours discussing classes and organising training workshops together.

A new life in Greenwich Point, Sydney

During my marriage, my husband wasn't supportive about yoga teaching at all. One morning I remember being neatly dressed, holding a little briefcase in my hand, ready to go out, and he asked where I was going. When I told him that I was applying for some yoga work, he just sneered at me. It took me a while, but I finally left my husband in 1973, two years after I taught my first yoga client.

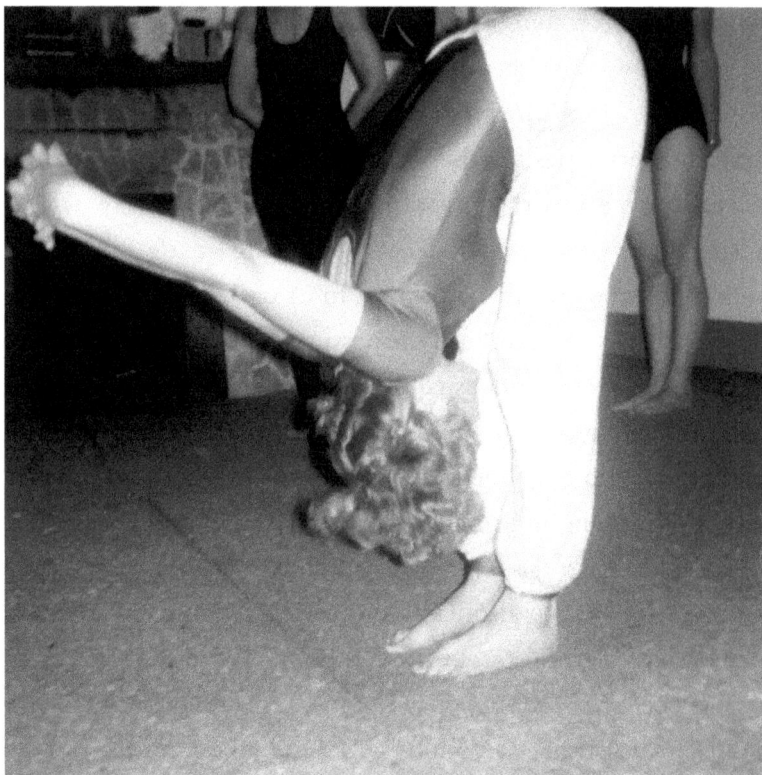

Maggie teaching a yoga class at Greenwich Point, 1980

The change in my circumstances worked out well. At that time, we had two young children, (now they are aged in their fifties and I also have great-grandchildren), and I rented a house at Greenwich Point in Sydney. Every window opened to a fabulous view of Lane Cove River where it enters Sydney Harbour. But it was a little old house and falling to bits! When I moved in, I had to get rid of the cobwebs, paint the house and fill in all the holes in the floors.

The owner of the house was an old woman, who lived upstairs, and I only had access to the downstairs part of the house, but that kept the rent very low for me. The lounge room became my yoga space and was soon filled with wall-to-wall yoga mats! I started teaching about six evening yoga classes a week. I remember a group of young men from Sydney University coming to my classes via the ferry; they thought yoga was quite a trendy thing to do. During winter I kept a log fire burning and students would collect wood for me on the way to class.

As well as teaching yoga at night, during the day I worked in the office of a television industry club in Sydney. My mother was secretary to the manager there, and I started helping out in the office, as well as in the dining room when it became busy. In the end I did every job that needed doing in the club.

That was my new life after marriage – and it was wonderful!

Have yoga mat will travel

While I was working at the television club, one of the guys there suggested that I apply for a job teaching yoga on cruise ships. Initially I didn't like the idea at all, but after some thought I decided to apply, and was accepted as a yoga teacher with Chandris Line (the Greek cruise ship company). The prospect of sailing between Greece and Australia was hugely appealing, and at that time I was also interested in Greek language, culture and art; I'd done some study in these topics at university as a mature-age student, when I was still married.

After my time with Chandris, I went on to work for CTC, SITMAR and P&O. I ended up teaching yoga on cruise ships for

15 years! They were always short cruises, about 10 days at a time, and I joined two or three each year. I chose the shorter cruises so I wasn't away from home for too long, and that meant I could also keep my yoga classes going in Sydney. I used fill-in teachers while I was away. At first, working on the cruise ships was fun: I made lots of new friends and travelled to different parts of the world – all very exciting. But after doing the same trips over and over again, I became quite blasé and bored with cruising. So, after 15 years I decided I'd had enough and quit. I still had my yoga classes running in Sydney and was also teaching widely across Sydney, getting to classes on buses and trains. In addition, I taught classes at home in Greenwich for two mornings and three evenings each week.

Ickwell Bury and Yoga for Health

Eventually I had to move out of the house at Greenwich, because the old lady who owned the property died and the house was being sold. At that stage, in the mid-1980s, I planned to live overseas to experience what it was like to be more of an 'international' person. I decided on visiting England first, to become a residential teacher for the Yoga for Health Foundation. The headquarters was in an old rented manor house called Ickwell Bury, located in rural Bedfordshire, near a town called Biggleswade. Aren't the names gorgeous?

Following that, my plan was to teach English language classes in Greece. I also arranged with a dance centre in Athens to teach tap dance classes and yoga when the new season started later in the year. Everything was organised for my voyage and my daughter and her fiancé came to see me off. As I was on the verge of departure, my daughter said, 'Oh mum, I think I'm pregnant.' Well, what a surprise! I still boarded the boat but decided not to stay away too long. In the end, I just went for a few months, to spend time at Ickwell Bury, until my first grandchild was born.

The centre at Ickwell Bury was a wonderful place and attracted people from around the world, many of whom suffered from chronic illnesses, including multiple sclerosis, cancer and arthritis. Ickwell Bury also had a kitchen garden with fresh, organic vegetables prepared daily for the residents' meals. Most of the staff were volunteers who received meals in exchange for their work.

I lived at Ickwell Bury for a couple of months teaching yoga to people with special needs – and it was a truly delightful experience. Specifically, I enjoyed meeting up with other people who were doing similar things: even if they were not teaching yoga, they were on the same wavelength. During my time there I met up with Michael Volin (who, I mentioned previously, was the brother of Nicolas, my first yoga teacher). I found Michael to be highly spiritual and he loved meditation in particular, compared to Nicolas, who seemed perhaps more physically inclined in the way he taught yoga.

During my time at Ickwell Bury I became deeply imbued with the energy around Yoga for Health, and upon returning to Australia, I realised that I'd 'let go' of my ego – this altered the way I taught yoga forever.

Bribie: my special island home

Throughout my life I was never influenced by making money; I just followed my heart and did what I was inspired to do. After I'd settled back into life in Australia, my mother died and left me a small amount of money. I hoped to buy a house with this inheritance. I had re-partnered and we were planning to move to Queensland together, in part because it was cheaper to buy housing there than in Sydney. But in the end my partner got cold feet (he was a lot younger than me) so I ended up going to Queensland alone. I was curious to see Bribie Island because I remembered that my father used to mention Bribie Island to us as children, describing how lovely it was.

After arriving in Brisbane, I caught the bus to Bribie Island, which is connected to the mainland by a bridge. I had very few belongings with me, as I'd been staying in youth hostels in Brisbane. I asked the bus driver if there was a local real estate agent on Bribie and he kindly dropped me at one in Bellara. And funnily enough, that's where I ended up living.

The real estate agent showed me through two houses, one of which had instant appeal: it had a large studio room with a lovely polished floor. I thought, *I can see myself teaching yoga here.*

So, I moved to Bribie Island and started classes in my own home at Bellara. That was 30 years ago. I taught classes every morning, and at lunch time I would walk down to the beach to eat my lunch and breathe in the fresh sea air. In the afternoons, I'd unpack a few more boxes to settle into my lovely island home. The old house needed quite a lot of repairs, so I put any money I made though teaching into maintaining the house. Luckily, one of the neighbours was a handyman and took on the repairs.

As soon as I'd settled in, I started driving down to Brisbane to attend a few classes: belly dancing, tap dancing, and finishing the art certificate course I'd previously started in Sydney, along with Greek language classes (at the Greek Club in West Brisbane). About three years later my aforementioned boyfriend, who was originally meant to move with me to Queensland, turned up at Bribie Island. My life changed once he moved in, and eventually I sold the house so we could buy a place in Brisbane together. Unfortunately, once again our relationship didn't work out, and 12 months later I returned to Bribie on my own. I guess it was 'meant to be' because I love living on Bribie and teaching yoga there.

How I became Swami Mrdukananda

During my time in Queensland, I sometimes ran yoga workshops up in Cairns and afterwards I'd head to Port Douglas to stay in the caravan park there for a short holiday. On one occasion I decided to visit Atherton instead, and when I was looking for some yoga classes to attend during my time there, I stumbled across a Sunday workshop with Swamiji Kamala-Mata Aranya.[14] The Aranya order dates back to ancient times but has been gradually updated over time to meet the demands of the modern world. Members strive to conduct their lives without causing harm or suffering to others; they also believe that tolerance of other people's philosophical and religious beliefs is essential. There is no insistence on following a vegetarian diet. I was a vegetarian for a while but became anaemic through the lack of iron in my diet; I had no energy and would often fall asleep during the day. These days I don't eat much meat but I do include a little chicken or sliced turkey to give my body some protein, which I find difficult as I don't particularly like it. I suppose I'm what you might call a 'lazy' vegetarian!

Anyway, after attending that initial Sunday workshop, I visited the Atherton Tablelands every time I was in Cairns and spent the day with members of the Aranya order. They were a very special group of people and I valued being a part of their community. After many visits, they invited me to become a Swami, and when I agreed to go through the initiation ritual, Swamiji Kamala-Mata Aranya said to me, 'At last. You are much loved in this neck of the woods dear Swami-to-be!'

Swamiji also told me that before anyone was initiated it would take her a whole week of meditating all night long to find the right name to give. The Sanskrit name she gave me was Swami Mrdukananda, which means 'gentle spiritual bliss'.

My personal joys and challenges with teaching yoga

I've been practising yoga for nearly 50 years now, and the thing I still enjoy most about teaching is sharing the philosophy of yoga with my students. I believe it's important to include this aspect in class because yoga is more than just postures and breathing exercises – it goes much deeper. I love structuring and preparing classes to give students an experience of yoga's depths, and I especially enjoy working with the *chakras* (the energy centres in the body). For many years I was a tutor on the remedial training courses for Yoga for Health in Australia. Although I don't do that anymore, I still run my own yoga workshops a couple of times each year on Bribie Island.

Another aspect of teaching that I really enjoy is seeing the way people look after class: much more relaxed, happier and younger! The other remarkable thing is that yoga helps everyone – teachers *and* students – to find their 'real' selves under all the layers. That's very special.

Some groups are more difficult to teach yoga to than others. In the past, high school students were my biggest challenge! I taught yoga classes in a block of weeks, or for the whole school term. In some classes, the students clearly enjoyed their practice and that was satisfying for me. But many students would just talk and laugh, and their behaviour was sometimes offensive with rude comments. 'Oh Miss, will you do that pose again for us?' came one boy's cheeky retort. He was referring to downward dog which I was demonstrating back-to-front, with my back facing the class.

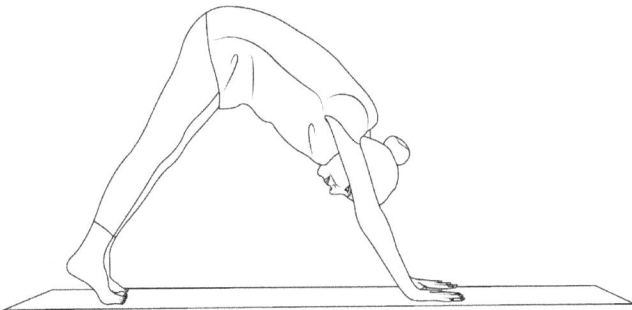

While adolescents have much to gain from yoga, approaches that work in classes with adults and children may not always be appropriate for them, and some modifications may need to be made.

I also taught yoga for pregnancy, and that was challenging in a different way. As a teacher, one has to be very careful with pregnant students, and classes need to be smaller than general yoga classes. Also, the class groups can't stay together because the women leave at different times to have their babies. They still do connect with each other in class and yoga often becomes a social event as well, but once they have their babies obviously it's difficult for them to get back to class for a period of time. Then another lot of new prenatal students start. So, there's a lot of coming and going. In spite of this inconsistency, I really enjoyed teaching yoga for pregnancy.

Teaching yoga on cruise ships also had its challenges — especially doing balance poses on rocky boats — but it was loads of fun!

Like all teachers, getting to class sometimes is difficult if I'm unwell or if something challenging is happening in my personal life. And when you're the only person teaching, it can be hard to take time off. In my case, I teach all year round, except for taking a break for a couple of weeks at Christmas.

Today, more than ever, I feel that to cultivate peace of mind, people need to practise yoga. Even the children I've taught often have very stiff bodies, but once they attend classes regularly their bodies start to loosen up. In yoga there is the old adage: 'A *flexible body leads to a flexible mind*'. So, practising yoga leads to a different way of thinking about life, and assists in moving people out of habitual, unhelpful patterns of behaviour. Over the years, when I've personally experienced certain problems, I've modified my teaching and home practice to accommodate my needs. At the same time, this wisdom has helped me to become more aware of my students' issues in class. To be honest, I especially enjoy teaching people who have health problems – when they take up remedial yoga practices you soon notice positive change.

The other day someone said to me, 'You shouldn't exercise before going to bed.' But that's when I like to do my yoga practice, and it's often the only time I have available. Recently I had a hip replacement operation and I'm still not comfortable getting up and down from the floor. So, to modify my practice, I've developed a little remedial yoga routine to do on the bed. I probably get the most benefit from *marjariasana* (cat pose), because it keeps my back supple and stretches out my fingers, which is excellent for arthritis. And every morning I practise my *pranayama* outdoors. Of course, I'm lucky on Bribie Island because the air is so clean for breathing practices.

Even when it's difficult to get to class, I keep on teaching because I enjoy it so much – it's one of the highlights of my week! After my earlier relationship problems, these days I have a companion who's genuinely interested in what I do; he's extremely helpful and morally supportive, as are my beautiful daughters (who both practise yoga, by the way).

Yoga has helped me get through many difficult times in my life, such as leaving my husband and losing my mother – it helped me get through it all and I'm so thankful that I found yoga all those years ago. As Swamiji used to say: '*Yoga lets the light shine.*'

REFLECTIONS

Maggie and I met up in the local village café after her yoga class. The café is also a nursery outlet so we sat outside amongst the trees, plants and garden paraphernalia. Coming from the southern winter, I revelled in the warm sunshine of a typical Queensland day. With a twinkle of humour playing across her face, Maggie confessed she had forgotten I was coming to interview her, at least until she received my reminder SMS on her mobile phone the day before. From my point of view that was perfect, because it meant there wasn't time for her to prepare. The interview flowed: it was like two old friends having a chat about yoga. Maggie's sense of humour, joy in life and passion for anything to do with yoga shone through. She told me her life was almost back to normal following her hip replacement operation in late 2016. Recently she started tap dancing again and has also resumed teaching Greek dancing for the University of the Third Age.

She explained that she spends a lot of time preparing her yoga classes. 'I think you're either a fusspot or you're not,' she said, 'and I'm a fusspot when it comes to my classes.' Maggie now teaches a 90-minute yoga class twice weekly, but it takes her half a day in real time to give a class due to her extensive preparation beforehand. Firstly, she works out what she's going to teach during the class and also looks through the attendance list to remind herself who is coming and what their conditions are. Then she might look for a book to quote from or develop a theme or something special to talk about in class. Finally, she told me that she likes to arrive at the venue early and put on the heaters or fans, so the room is cosy or cool, as needed, by the time the students arrive. All this preparation and care for her students shows in the quality of her teaching. The class I attended was a truly beautiful therapeutic session.

The time flew, and as I drove on to Caboolture to meet with Vivian Vieritz (who features in the next chapter), I pondered over Maggie's wisdom. I recalled attending some yoga classes where teachers taught, calling out instructions, with their eyes closed throughout the class, appearing oblivious to the need to safeguard their charges in front of them. But Maggie didn't close her eyes. There is a lot to be said for the value of thorough training and support provided through organisations like Yoga for Health, and for lifelong learning and ongoing curiosity about yoga.

Maggie's experience with anaemia also resonated with me. Like her, I've committed to eating a vegetarian diet over the years. But despite carefully planning a balanced diet I have developed debilitating anaemia – with my doctors advising me that for my health I need to include at least some animal protein in my diet. So, for me it's been a lesson about learning to exist in my body, regardless of my beliefs.

A few weeks later, I received a wonderful package of goodies from Maggie in the mail. It included a series of photos all carefully labelled with headings and dates, including information about Yoga for Health. Until I met Maggie I'd never heard of Yoga for Health or the training courses they offered. This movement has produced a wonderful legacy of remedial yoga teachers like Maggie, remaining devoted to yoga, assisting students to optimise their health, being committed to lifelong learning, and having compassion for all people. As Maggie said: yoga was her best option – it has helped her to accept the unchangeable with grace and serenity, and to transform rocky moments into periods of growth.

#3
VIVIAN VIERITZ

～✦～

YOU'RE NEVER TOO OLD
TO PRACTISE YOGA

Don't ever let anyone tell you that you can't do something new

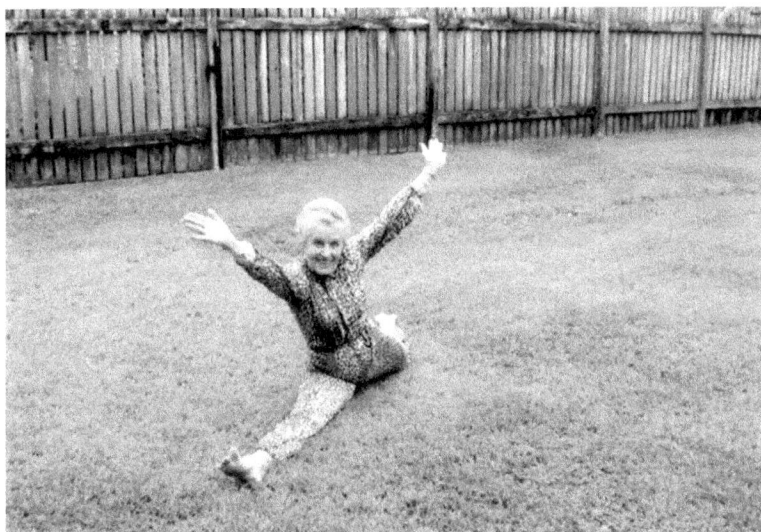

Vivian on her 90th birthday

Here is
Vivian
In her ninety-sixth year,
Still strong and teaching yoga.
Age is no barrier
To headstand
For her!

At the age of 95, Vivian teaches one yoga class a week to around 18 students at the Caboolture Community Centre, in Queensland. As with the other yoga teachers featured in this book, I arranged to attend Vivian's class before we did the interview. However, these plans went awry. After arriving on the Sunshine Coast, I tried calling her landline numerous times to re-confirm our arrangements, receiving what sounded like an engaged signal. In the end, I decided to go along to Vivian's regular Monday evening yoga class – but no-one turned up except me! I thought: 'Oh, I hope Vivian's all right; I wonder why the class isn't on.'

The next day, when I managed to track Vivian down, she was in the middle of moving to a unit in supported care, which explained why her phone was disconnected. It was a busy time so she had cancelled her yoga classes for a couple of weeks. I laughed when, with a smile in her voice, she said to me, 'I have to write your phone number down in lipstick dear because with the move I can't find a pen.' Later the same day, we sat side-by-side on Vivian's bed in her new unit looking through lots of wonderful photos, many of them black and white snapshots taken before colour photography was common. Spread out on the bed they were like a rich decoupage displaying Vivian's memoirs.

Yoga is Vivian's first love but her other passions are square dancing and ballroom dancing. In 2003, she was Belle of the Ball at Caboolture. Despite the upheaval of moving, Vivian was planning to attend square dancing that evening because (as she explained) she could just turn up, choose to sit one set out, or do the next if she wanted to. Like yoga it was fun, but without the added responsibility of preparing and teaching a class.

Vivian's many words of wisdom to me during our session included: 'Don't ever let anyone tell you that you can't do something new – you just need to try.' I also received invaluable instruction in how to do a headstand pose safely. Vivian and I moved down onto the floor and practised together. She emphasised the correct placement of my hands, arms and elbows, showing me how to make a little cup with my hands, with elbows pointing slightly out, chin tucked in and the crown of my head placed in my hands. As we finished the pose she added: 'Take notice of how I've instructed you when you do headstand next time and you'll always be safe.' And I thought to myself, 'Yes, I will.'

Here's more of what Vivian had to say about her lifelong journey with yoga.

VIVIAN'S STORY

A long lifetime of loving yoga

I was born in Toowoomba and raised in a family of seven children: four girls and three boys, but I'm the only one who teaches yoga. I started practising yoga at the age of six, but what I did then wasn't known as yoga; it was simply called 'exercise'. As a child, I loved performing cartwheels and handstands. It didn't matter where I was, if I saw a wall I would immediately tuck my dress inside my bloomers, throw my hands down to the ground and *up* my legs would go. My mother used to say to me, 'Vivian, as soon as I'd see you take your hands towards your head, I knew what was coming next; I'd walk away and try to disown you!'

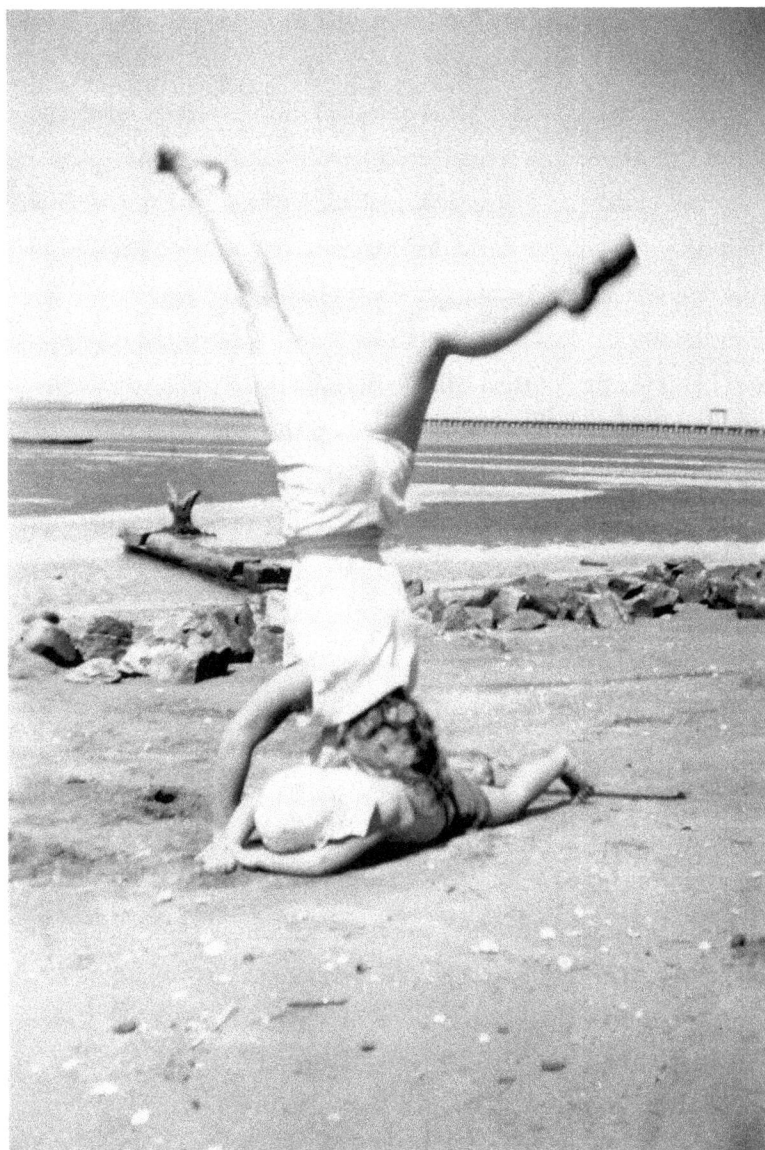

Vivian aged 27 doing a handstand over her son Larry

When I was six, my family moved to Sydney and I spent my early childhood years there.

Although I always practised yoga, I didn't start teaching until after I married and returned to Queensland with my husband and two children. At that stage, I didn't know anyone who was involved in yoga, but I decided I wanted to become a yoga teacher one day. My motto in life has always been: *'You learn by doing.'* I didn't have a teacher to train me and there wasn't a special teacher training course available in those days, so I simply started teaching yoga on my own. We lived on the coast at Coolum and I taught five classes a week there. At first, I called my classes 'light exercise' because yoga was virtually unknown in Queensland at the time.

I remember being inspired by watching Roma Blair on television in the 1960s when she presented her yoga program, *Relaxing with Roma*. For those who haven't heard of her, Roma Blair was one of the early pioneers of yoga in Australia. Before her program started, few people in Australia had heard about yoga and she promoted it to a wide audience. Roma also advanced yoga through setting up a professional organisation for yoga teachers in 1967: the International Yoga Teachers Association (IYTA), and I joined soon after it commenced. Over the years, I became fairly well acquainted with Roma, because when I went down to attend yoga activities in Sydney she was always there.

I was inspired by several other yoga teachers whose classes and workshops I attended over the years. My teacher in Coolum, Elsa Rabold, escaped with her husband from East Germany after World War Two, and they migrated to Australia in the 1950s. As a child in Germany, Elsa had learnt yoga in primary school where it was called 'floor exercises'. In Australia, she taught yoga classes in a hall at Nambour (near her house in Mapleton). A few years after I'd shifted to Coolum, one of the students who came to my exercise classes phoned me to say, 'I've just heard there's a lady who teaches Iyengar Yoga in Nambour. How about we go and try it?' So, off we went to Elsa's class. That was my first experience with an Iyengar teacher – and I loved it. I think it must have been serendipity because Elsa's lease on the hall in Nambour expired the very same night we attended her class. I said to my student, 'How about we ask Elsa if she'll come to Coolum to teach yoga?'

So, that's how Elsa's classes came to Coolum, where I learnt from her all the Iyengar poses and how to teach yoga properly. It was due to Elsa that I was able to teach a better class.

How to hold poses for maximum benefits

Given Elsa Rabold's influence, the way I teach yoga leans towards the Iyengar style. I've observed that the major difference between Iyengar and other types of yoga is that when you perform a posture with Iyengar, you *hold* it. These days, the latest fashion is to practise yoga in a flow, moving through one pose after another in quick succession. For me this feels wrong because I believe you get the most benefit from holding each posture. For example, if you perform a side twist quickly: turning the upper body to the right, then immediately rotating to the left, then returning to the centre – what good does it do? Perhaps it provides a tiny stretch, but the body has no real time to benefit.

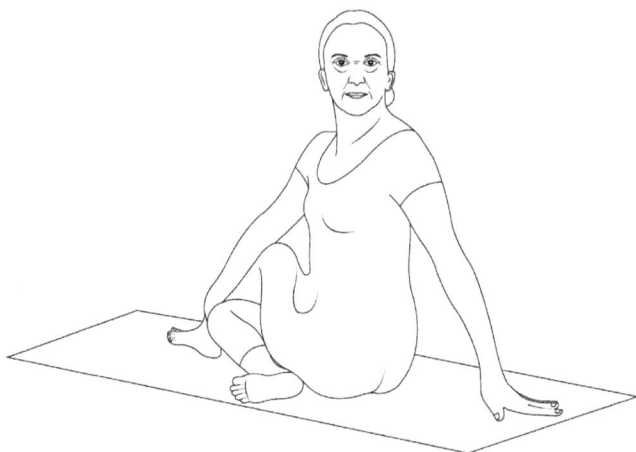

How to twist properly: The first thing I teach before moving into a twist is to take a deep breath in and lengthen up through the whole spine, while keeping the shoulders relaxed and away from the ears. Lengthening, twisting and holding the position for a few breaths: what a difference these three stages make, rather than just turning from side to side. The after-effect is magnificent! This is what I have always done, in my personal practice and in teaching classes. To me, this is the secret of teaching yoga and I believe that many teachers just don't know about it. Of course, it's only my opinion but try experimenting yourself doing poses involving twists. First go in and out of a twist quickly and then try my way: lengthening, twisting and holding for a few breaths on each side, and compare the difference in how you feel afterwards.

My teaching style

I used to teach two-hour classes, but these days I teach for just one and a half hours. Maybe I'm getting older and a bit lazier! Looking back, I'm quite sure my students never minded doing two hours of yoga. During my classes, there is no lying down for a long relaxation at the beginning. I want the students to use their muscles, not to think, *Oh, I'm relaxed now and don't feel like doing any work.* They do get a short relaxation at the end of class, where the focus is on releasing the muscles they've been using and switching off their mental chatter. What I often say during relaxation is something like: 'Let everything go, all the muscles you've been using . . . feel as though they are floating away from you.' As a teacher, you don't want students so relaxed that they're driving home, half-asleep in traffic. Maybe it's not a problem in little Caboolture, because there isn't much traffic, but imagine driving home in Sydney!

When I teach, I always wear leotards and tights, so the students can see how my body moves as I demonstrate poses. If a teacher dresses in baggy pants, what can the students see? They can't observe how the teacher's legs or knees are moving, or how the muscles are working. And demonstrating like this is the best way for students to learn yoga. Although I lean toward Iyengar-style teaching, where the use of props like bolsters and straps is common, in my opinion the average person does not require them. What happens when students decide to practise at home and don't have any props to rely on? However, if a student in class really feels the need for a prop, such as a block, then I'm fine with it. For my classes, the only essential item is a mat; I use two mats together, with one thicker than the other. Finding the right mat, which is not too thick or thin, depends on the type of floor practised on, and also individual needs. Knees in particular are highly vulnerable to injury on hard floors. If you are new to yoga I advise a thick mat; try it out and if you feel comfortable practising on it, then it should be suitable.

I will continue to teach yoga for as long as I can, because I love it and believe it's what I'm meant to do in my life. And yoga keeps me healthy as well as benefiting my students. At one time I did consider giving up because I'm definitely not as good at yoga as I once was, but my students asked me to keep teaching them.

So, I said to them, 'Well, as long as you don't mind me making mistakes – or if I get stuck for words, helping me out?'

'Oh no, we don't mind!' they replied.

This wonderful support is one of the reasons why teaching yoga is worthwhile. When I left Coolum to move to Caboolture my students cried and I hated leaving them. I remember one student saying goodbye as tears welled up in her eyes, and as she hurried away, she turned back to face me and said, 'Vivian, I'm a better person for having known you.' You can't get a better compliment than that – it was such a lovely thing to say. And three women I taught are now yoga teachers themselves, which is another rewarding aspect of teaching for so many years.

I have no idea what other teachers charge these days but my yoga class costs five dollars, and it has for a long time. I want everyone to come whether they can afford to or not. Over the past 60 years, I haven't kept a single cent of the earnings from my classes. I've donated the money to various charities, who keep me updated as to how they are progressing with curing different cancers, such as breast, prostate and children's cancer – and it's truly heartening for me to know this.

Practising inverted poses safely

Without a doubt, my favourite pose is the headstand, but it's important to perform it correctly. I always make sure my head is comfortable and my neck is safe. When I'm in the headstand, I often feel so comfy that I close my eyes and could almost fall asleep! If you practise the headstand correctly, you'll never hurt yourself, but it's an advanced pose with a number of precautions, and therefore unsuitable for the average student. So, I never teach the headstand in a general yoga class; it's only suitable if students are strong enough and have practised yoga for a long time.

Another important factor with the headstand is a willingness for the students to learn and follow instructions; as a teacher, you really don't want students doing their own thing when you're trying to teach this pose. Students often have no idea of the precision involved, or what to do with their hands, or how to position their elbows and arms. And the neck in headstand is extremely vulnerable; it terrifies me looking at the amount of pressure this pose can exert on some students' necks. What happens if an inexperienced student attempts the headstand at home without the guidance of a proper teacher? In my view it risks drastic consequences.

It's also important to remember that there are many other wonderful inverted poses that people can do, such as the shoulder stand – although they still need to take care and observe the safety measures for practising it. For instance, it's important to ensure that the head stays aligned, as well as using an appropriate amount of padding under the shoulders for support. Some students can overdo things with inverted poses, but fortunately the majority are sensible.

A special compliment from Mr Iyengar

I met Mr Iyengar[15] the first time he visited Australia in 1983. People came from far and wide to attend his yoga workshop, which was held in an enormous hall in Sydney. He was walking around amidst the crowd of participants when he said, 'If you can do a headstand then perform one now.' And along he went from one person to the next calling out, 'You call that a headstand? Ha, look at that shoulder! Oh, look how this arm is positioned.' He was disgusted with the quality of headstands.

Then Mr Iyengar announced, 'Those who can do a proper headstand, come up onto the stage now and show me.'

I thought to myself, *Well, I know I can do the headstand – but can I do it properly?*

My yoga mat was right at the back of the hall and by the time I reached the stage I was almost last in line. Mr Iyengar was moving along the stage criticising people's headstands. As he came towards me, I felt a little panic rise up inside, *What is he going to say about me?*

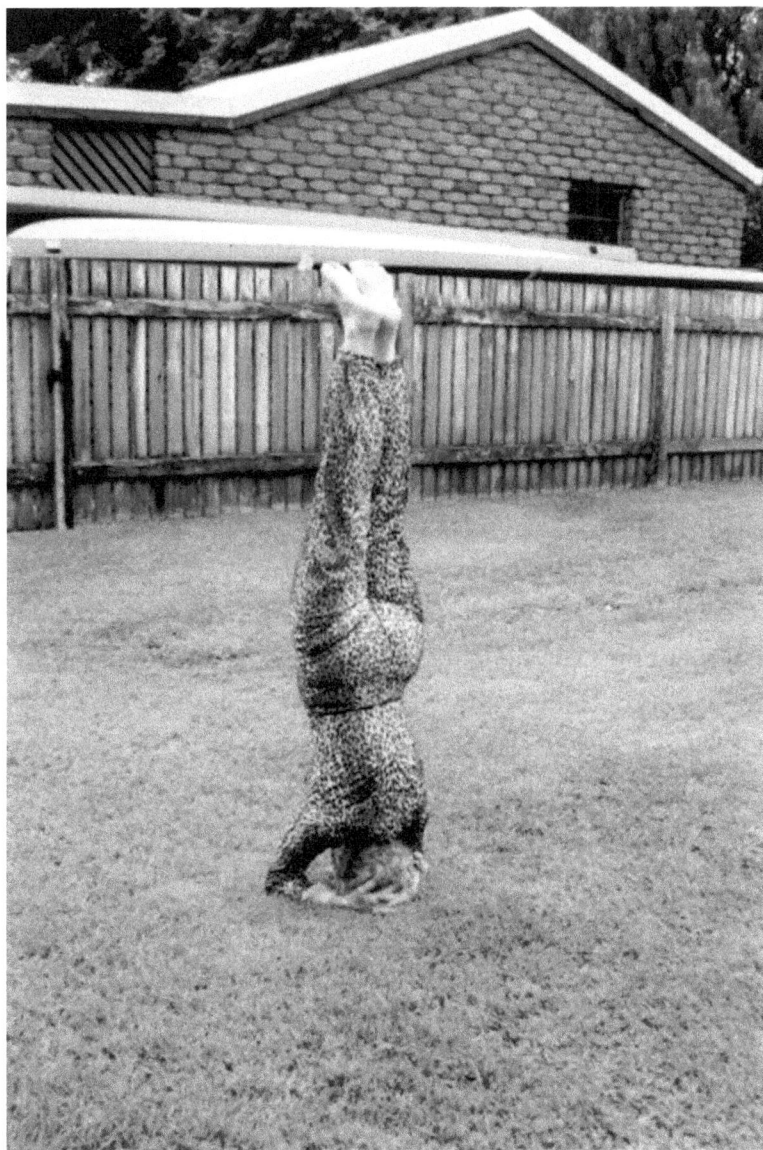

Vivian in her favourite pose, the headstand

I went up into the headstand and thought, *Gee, am I doing it properly?*

Then I heard Mr Iyengar say, 'Well, at last we have a decent headstand!'

I nearly fell out of my headstand with shock! It was *my* headstand he was praising. A compliment from Mr Iyengar compares to winning the Golden Casket (Lotto) at least ten times, and that's no exaggeration because Mr Iyengar rarely gave compliments. After the workshop, many people said to me, 'What did you do to deserve that? Fancy getting a compliment from Mr Iyengar!' And until that moment I didn't realise I could do a perfect headstand. So, that's the story of my special experience with Mr Iyengar, and all these years later I still can't get over it.

Mr Iyengar was a great teacher. He passed away in 2014. He was about the same age as me and I thought he would live forever. So many people live to 100 these days, and I was surprised when I read that he had died because he was such an extraordinary person, and I really believed he would live for a lot longer.

Coping with life's changes

My husband, Arnold Vieritz, had been a sergeant major in the army. He was six foot one in height, compared to my tiny four foot eleven and a half inches. Arnold was never interested in yoga, but was genuinely happy that I practised it. Sadly, I lost my dear husband over 30 years ago when he had a massive heart attack in Coolum. After he died, I never met anyone else I wanted to share the rest of my life with.

In the years that followed, I was living alone in Coolum when my eyesight started to deteriorate. Back in those days, Coolum only had two little shops and there were no buses, which meant I had to drive to a larger town to do the shopping. I decided to move to Caboolture, so that if I lost my sight completely, I wouldn't need to drive (as the shops and other facilities would be close by). It's not obvious by looking at me today, but I only have sight in one eye. My grandmother had a crossed eye and guess who inherited it? My eye was crossed for all my early years of teaching, even when I did the headstand for Mr Iyengar. It was finally corrected 23 years ago, after I moved to Caboolture. I had an operation for cataracts as well, and a special lens was put into the eye. This meant I didn't have to wear glasses, which I was thrilled about, because I have a small face and glasses don't suit me.

So, losing my husband, having cataracts, and sight in only one eye, were the circumstances that led me to live in Caboolture. Another factor, which influenced me to move, was that as soon as you teach yoga in a place, you make new friends. But even today, I still love Coolum and feel sorry I don't live there anymore. In hindsight, if I'd known the cataract operation was going to be so successful, I wouldn't have moved. But at my age you can't start again somewhere else. I'm not 21 anymore! Well, in truth you *can* start again, but I wouldn't like to leave behind my wonderful group of yoga students in Caboolture.

Now I've moved to my unit in supported care because I'm 95 and getting towards the 100-year mark, and my son has been worried about me living alone. Sometimes I forget certain things

— where I put this or that object — whereas at other times my memory is perfect. Now with shifting to a new unit, I can't find anything! My daughter lives in Indonesia and wanted to fly over and help me pack for the move, but my son helped me; luckily, he's doing the bulk of it as I couldn't have managed it by myself. At the moment, I've only half-moved in as my old unit is still full of my belongings. My new unit is much smaller and I should have said, 'no, no, no' instead of 'yes, yes, yes' when we sorted the items! I still have to finish going through my clothes — there are *so* many. Your clothing collection soon builds up when you have square dancing outfits, ballroom dancing costumes, yoga garments and normal attire. What's left after I finish sorting will be donated to the opportunity shop where my daughter-in-law works. I don't mind my bits and pieces going to an op shop because somebody will benefit from them, but I'd be very upset to see my things thrown into a dump.

Yoga for ongoing physical and mental health

Yoga incorporates all a person needs for keeping the body and mind healthy — this is why I believe in it so much. The most important aspect of yoga is the breathing practice, because the majority of people just don't breathe properly. When I ask students in my classes *where* they breathe, most of them point to their chests and say, 'I breathe up here.' I want them to learn how to breathe into the belly. Watch a baby breathe — what a lovely demonstration of our natural breath.

Other important benefits of yoga come through the twisting

and stretching poses; I also believe that inverted poses are valuable, but certainly never on a full stomach – that's taboo! As I mentioned previously, headstands are not suitable for everyone, but good old shoulder stands are accessible for most people, and a great way for tipping the body upside down and getting the benefits that go with inversions.

The idea of *use it or lose it* I hold absolutely true, because I don't know of anyone else my age who is as healthy as me. Apart from regular check-ups to make sure everything is fine, I seldom visit the doctor. A few years ago, my local doctor told me I had osteoporosis due to being fair-skinned and having low vitamin D levels. When I visited the medical specialist about my condition he said, 'With your bone density I expected you to arrive in a wheelchair!'

My bones might be weak but my muscles hold everything together. I'm so glad that I kept on practising yoga for all these years. And my blood pressure is classed as high, but not dangerously high. This doesn't affect me because I've had high blood pressure for years. Perhaps the reason it's high is because I'm the sort of person who is constantly on the go and I've been like this all my life. By the age of 95, most people would probably have high blood pressure; it just doesn't make any difference to me – I still stand on my head!

I don't attend other yoga teachers' classes anymore. I do my own practice and teach one class a week. I practise whenever I feel like it, which is not every day. There is no need to, because after so many years of practising yoga I've kept my body lengthened. People who don't practise yoga tend to sit with the pelvis tucked under and lower back slumped, which is detrimental for spinal health. No matter where I go, or who I'm with, I make sure I sit up straight with spine lengthened, tummy tucked in, and shoulders drawn slightly back (not *right* back because it would look odd). It's actually easy to sit like this, and if you practise it every day, your body will stay straight and strong, because you are *using* it.

Attitude and gratitude

I call 'attitude' my magic word because it is truly your attitude towards life that counts. If you have the right attitude, you'll cope with whatever life dishes out. Pause for a moment and think about this. Some people have lives where they experience one tragedy after another, yet they're the happiest, most contented people you'll ever meet. Then you have the opposite situation, where people have all they need and life is running smoothly; in spite of this, they hate everybody, including themselves, and also what they do to earn a living.

Certainly, yoga helps with developing a different attitude and accepting the circumstances of your life. I love all the things I've done in my life. I went to Europe to do square dancing and visited India several times; once was to visit Mr Iyengar, which seems like a long time ago now. Another time, I travelled to India with my sister, Shirley Thoms. When Shirley was 16, she became the first female vocalist to record country music in Australia. From then on, she was nicknamed 'Australia's Yodelling Sweetheart'. As an adult she developed Parkinson's disease and wanted me to take her to visit the famous healer, Sai Baba. We went to India, and sat with a crowd of people as Sai Baba walked amongst us. Everyone was given strict orders not to touch him – but somebody *did* – and he was furious! Unfortunately, Shirley didn't receive a cure in India for her Parkinson's, and she died in 1999 from complications of the disease. I believe nobody heals you, except yourself. Shirley wasn't interested in following yoga, and if people are not open to it (even if it *is* your own family) you can't persuade them to do something they don't want to do.

My children could have come to my yoga classes but they weren't interested either. Their attitude has always been: 'Yoga is good for you mum, as long as you don't want us to do it.' And I understand this because yoga really is about *me*, and I'm the one who wants to keep practising it.

For my 95th birthday (on 12th March 2017) I attended a power yoga retreat on Stradbroke Island (in Queensland). Tammy Williams[16] at Yoga NRG invited me, and she organised everything for the whole weekend, including the boat trip to get there. The other participants were amazed when I did every class with them. They just couldn't believe that tiny little me, at my age, could do hard yoga postures *and* hold them. The retreat was just magic – it was so lovely of Tammy to give me this precious gift for my birthday.

I think I'm the luckiest person in the whole world because I'm 95 years old, healthy and still doing what I love – teaching my yoga.

REFLECTIONS

I felt honoured that Vivian had given me the gift of her time during a busy period in the middle of moving house. As she said, when we'd chatted on the phone earlier the same day: 'It's just a bad time, really, to catch up' – but catch up we did, and what a fun afternoon we had together.

I was amazed at how strong and flexible Vivian still is at the age of 95. She says it's because she holds the yoga poses in keeping with the strong Iyengar-style yoga she teaches. Vivian shared so many valuable tips about teaching yoga safely. This is precious knowledge that she has built up over many years of teaching. During our discussion about how to do a headstand safely she went up into the pose several times with ease. She also moved down onto and up from the floor with little effort, which is sometimes problematic for people half Vivian's age.

After our meeting, when I drove from Caboolture to my accommodation on Bribie Island, the sky was vivid with the colours of sunset, and the environment around was beginning to fall calm and silent. I thought about what a blissful afternoon it had been. I had really enjoyed talking with Vivian, experiencing her infectious laughter and joy of life, and hearing about the many friendships and social connections she still maintains across all age groups through keeping up her yoga teaching. And it is clear how truly connected she is with her local community.

I started planning when I could get back to the Sunshine Coast to do one of Vivian's yoga classes.

#4
ANITA CLARA

⟨∽⟩

CHANGING FROM THE INSIDE-OUT

As I age, yoga looks after my body ~ but meditation
takes me deeper into stillness

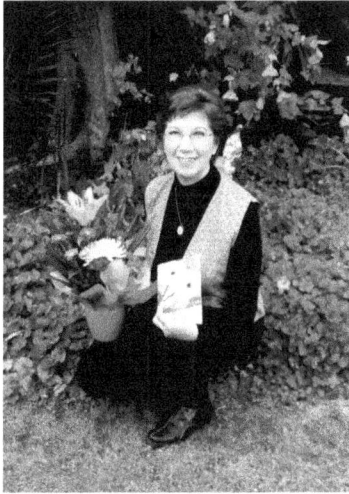

Anita in her garden

Here is
Anita,
A teacher always
Of Dru – yoga of the heart
And meditation.
Seeking truth
And light.

Nine years ago, I moved back to Adelaide from Melbourne, and was searching for a yoga class to attend when I stumbled across Anita's Dru meditation classes. From the first class it felt special; similar to several other forms of meditation, Dru meditation incorporates breath and body awareness. However, the rest of this class was quite different, beginning with preparatory work to relax the body and mind before meditation. Activations (limbering and warming up exercises) were followed by gentle yoga with special sequences designed to release blocked energy from the body. Next came the 'icing on the cake' – a scrumptious guided relaxation and finally, meditation.

As Anita says, Dru meditation and yoga cater to different body types and experience. Sitting quietly in calm meditation is comfy for some but unbearably painful for others. So, it's all about finding what works for you. If your hips are cranky, then it's perfectly acceptable – even advisable – to sit in a chair.

Anita is a perfect model for the benefits of the Dru practices. Passionate and enthusiastic, she exhibits a joy of life peppered with a delightful sense of humour. Being around her makes me think, 'I want what she has.'

We held the interview sitting in Anita's home office, looking out through the sliding glass door into her lush garden with its backdrop of treetop gums. Dappled winter sunlight struggled through the clouds that day, but we were warm and snug inside. With the abundance of trees, it felt as if I was in the middle of a tranquil woodland.

Unlike most of the other teachers featured in this book, Anita found meditation first and then came to yoga some years later.

She describes the meditation practices as transformative. In fact, after she had been meditating for a few years, one of her sons said to her, 'you're different'. When she asked him to describe what he meant, he added, 'you're calmer'.

In Anita's story, which follows, she recalls how her life 'pre-meditation and yoga' was very different to how it is now.

ANITA'S STORY

Getting my health 'back on track'

I didn't start yoga early in life; my yoga journey began in my mid-forties, when I needed to get my health back on track. I was a divorced, single parent working as a school teacher in Adelaide. For many years, I was employed under contracts, which involved working in numerous schools. Every time I started at a new school, I'd teach different courses, which meant reinventing the teaching programme all over again. Although I loved teaching, after 13 years, it really took its toll. One day I thought, *Oh my goodness, I'm spending my whole life just teaching and programming.*

By this time, I also felt profoundly tired. When I went to see a doctor about my flagging energy levels, she asked me all kinds of questions about my background to discover more about my life and what was happening to me. I was diagnosed with fibromyalgia and chronic fatigue, and also had a dangerous melanoma removed. Dr Miranda never made me feel as if I was making up the tiredness and chronic fatigue. She was a beautiful, compassionate person who got me back on track with my health. And she also asked if I'd ever tried meditation.

Although I was 45 at the time, I'd never heard the word 'meditation' before. So, I found a couple of books on meditation, one of which was by Ian Gawler.[17] I started using the techniques from his book and tried several different meditation groups. However, the groups were interested in psychic meditation with clairvoyance, which wasn't what I wanted – I needed to recover my health. So, I meditated by myself at home for up to four hours a day. Once I was meditating regularly, I found it hugely beneficial. Meditation was truly a gift because it made me pay attention to my body, to my illness, and to my physical behaviour, and it stopped me running around having a busy, stressful life, which allowed my body time to heal.

As I started to recover from my illness, I wanted to only work part-time. Three days a week would have been ideal, but then I was offered a full-time teaching position again, which I decided to accept. The first two days of term, before the kids came back to school, always consisted of planning. On the first day, I remember hearing the staff droning in the background about the same old issues: 'Behaviour management. What are we going to do with the curriculum? This is what the Department wants us to do!' I just sat there and blanked out. Later, when I had a cuppa with a friend, I said, 'I'm going to resign at the end of the term.'

My friend replied, 'Anita, it's only the first day back.'

'No, the kids weren't even at school today,' I said. 'It's not about the kids – it's about the unreasonable expectations the Department has for teachers.'

As soon as I'd made my decision to resign, I went to see the principal and he tried to talk me out of it. But meditation and my health were too important to me by then. The meditation practice had changed me from the inside out. I'd started to reclaim myself and felt a sense of completeness. It was almost as if I was looking at the world through new eyes. What I had considered important before was no longer important. At that point, I said to myself, *This term is going to be a time to see how well meditation is working in my life, and if I'm the person I need to be – balanced and still – then I can convey that to others without trying very hard at all, just through being who I am.* And that's exactly what happened. Even the children in my year three class noticed the difference – and my 'stillness' did have an impact on them. When I taught, I paused more often and didn't get upset if the children played up. I remember one morning, halfway through term, entering the classroom to find a new air-conditioning system plonked right in the middle of the carpet where the kids would sit for our morning talks. When the children arrived, they said, 'Miss Clara, what are we going to do? It's right in the middle of the room.'

'That's okay,' I replied, calmly. 'We'll go out to the oval and sit under a tree to have our morning talks. All right, everybody line up.'

We went outside and I experienced a deep awareness of just sitting on the earth with the group, feeling really grounded. The children waited for me to speak; I could see they were sensing something different about me. And instead of immediately saying, 'Okay, whose turn is it to talk?' I said, 'Isn't it nice being outside, sitting on the ground, underneath the shade of a tree.'

It was a defining moment for me, further reinforcing my decision, and at the end of term I left teaching.

Two of my background strengths as a school teacher were in curriculum writing and developing teaching programmes. So, I researched the topics of meditation and counselling, and created several stress management programmes to help people in need to get 'back on track'. People also started coming to me for one-on-one meditation sessions. I wasn't a trained counsellor at the time (that came later), but as a teacher I'd given a great deal of counselling to students, as well as parents. In addition, I'd attended the Pathways Program, which was a personal development course.

Discovering Dru: 'yoga of the heart'

After recovering from my various illnesses, I was extremely lethargic and needed to build muscular strength. I would often go for a walk down the street, but that would be it for my exercise. One day I was flicking through the Guardian Messenger (a local paper) and spotted a little ad from the Yoga Teachers Institute of South Australia (YTISA) promoting an 18-month teacher training course in Integral Yoga. There was a list of the topics and I noticed that meditation was included. Regarding yoga, I'd never practised it before and had absolutely no idea what it entailed, but deep down I knew I was going to do the course. I didn't have much money but enough came through from the programmes I was teaching at home, and luckily the training wasn't expensive.

This Integral Yoga teacher training course gave me a comprehensive background in yoga philosophy, and every aspect of the Eight Limbs of Yoga.[18] I thoroughly enjoyed the course and became quite entrenched in yoga, although I wasn't yet teaching it.

In 1998, while I was doing one of the Integral Yoga training modules, I was introduced to Dru Yoga.[19] It was sheer serendipity because the Dru teachers phoned the YTISA. 'We're from the UK,' they said, 'and teach Dru Yoga, which is *yoga of the heart* – would you be interested if we organised a session in Adelaide?'

At that time, no one had actually heard of Dru Yoga, because 1998 was the very first year these teachers came to Australia. Initially they ran a full day workshop (on a Sunday) at the Theosophical Society in Adelaide, which I attended. I found Dru Yoga remarkably different to the tradition I'd been training in, and the Dru teachers had a huge impact on me, because they taught from the heart – and there was a tangible feeling of this. I thought, *This yoga is perfect for me.* During the workshop, the teachers took us through not just the yoga practices, but also yoga's therapeutic aspects. And I immediately understood how useful this style of yoga was going to be for the work I was currently involved in. Dru Yoga was also softer on the body and exactly what I needed – instead of really strong postures. The Dru teachers wanted to do another workshop in Adelaide the following year and I organised a venue for them. That's how I became involved with the Dru yogis.

In 1999, I moved to country Victoria with my new partner. By then, I'd completed the Integral Yoga course and wanted to join the Dru teacher training, being held in New South Wales. But I was also thinking of the expense and wondering where the money would come from. Our move to Victoria was done on the cheap; we'd loaded my goods and chattels in a ute and driven all the way from Adelaide up through the Riverland to Robinvale. I remember feeling immensely relieved when the move was over. I'd taken all my essential items out of their boxes and was ready to lie down on the couch and enjoy a good read, when the phone rang. The caller was a beautiful lady from the Life Foundation (which is what Dru International was called in those days) who wanted to know if I was still interested in undertaking the teacher training course, as I'd previously expressed interest. That phone call was so timely – the very next day after my house sale had settled – so I agreed to do the course. I felt it was just meant to be.

At the time, I wasn't worried about how I was going to travel from my new place in the middle of nowhere (in country Victoria) to Kincumber in New South Wales, to attend the course. I soon found out it was incredibly complicated, but I was determined to get there. Eventually I worked out a travel plan: I drove to Mildura, which was one hour away (where Rex Airlines was located), then I flew to Melbourne, and from Melbourne to Sydney. From there I caught the train to Gosford, followed by a taxi to Kincumber. I did that journey many times over for the two and a half years duration of the course. It was the first yoga teacher course Dru ran internationally and I was one of the first teachers trained in Australia.

Yoga as a vessel for transformation

The majority of people practise yoga first, before moving on to meditation, but I was a solid meditator for two years before I attempted yoga. When I first started practising yoga, my body wasn't flexible at all; I had little glitches throughout my spine and joints, but through yoga they gradually disappeared. Yoga not only healed my body on a physical level, it penetrated the nooks and crannies of my being, and I found that it took away all the negative conditioning many of us grow up with. Once I experienced the benefits of daily yoga practice, I wanted to share what I had learnt with others. So, I started teaching yoga in a local school hall. At first, I taught in the tradition of Integral Yoga, but gradually my classes incorporated more of the Dru approach. Although I couldn't call myself a Dru teacher until I'd completed the training course, it was acceptable to call my classes 'Dru style yoga'. The amazing thing was that once I learnt something new in my Dru training, a student would come along to class who needed that specific practice. I remember thinking, *I've just learnt that, now I'm going to pass it on.*

If only one person turned up to class, which sometimes happened, I believed that person was vitally important and had come to my class for a reason. As a teacher, you ask yourself, *What can I provide to assist this person?* And the more I practised yoga and daily meditation, the more deeply I sensed this aspect. When I teach, I feel as if this person – the 'me' who exists in the physical world – is just a vessel to help others.

During my early years of teaching, I liked to plan the yoga

programme from week to week so I could decide, *Okay, I managed to introduce a bit of this practice last week, so do I want to go further or stick with it?'* As I grew in experience and my classes expanded, often when I stood up in front of the class, the planned programme was completely discarded. My students let me know in different ways what they needed. The philosophy of Dru Yoga fitted into the stress management and self-development programmes I'd been teaching like a 'hand in a glove' and it was hard to hold back my enthusiasm. I'd suggest things like, 'Would you like to try a little bit of movement and see how that helps?' Or ask, 'What kind of movement do you normally do in your everyday life?' Dru Yoga provided many tools that not only restored balance, health and wellness in my own life but also assisted so many other people in a gentle way. I set up a centre *Sundarra* at my home in Victoria. The whole focus was on helping people to develop themselves.

Over the years, I've taught a wide variety of people. I remember when a social worker hired me to introduce a four-week programme to teenage mums, who were aged 14 and 15, and they absolutely loved it. I also worked with older people in retirement villages; the nursing staff kept calling me back to teach what they called 'being in the moment' skills. Then they referred people to me for one-on-one sessions. I remember one lady who was afraid of standing after she'd had a bad fall. She found *yoga nidra* (deep relaxation) very helpful to alleviate her fear. We focused on relaxing each part of the body and being in the present moment.

Yoga is a vessel for transformation because a particular practice or move performed in a certain way will affect a specific part of the body, emotional state, or one's overall health. It is not simply a matter of the brain thinking, *Oh, I've done yoga, and now I feel great*. It's so much more than that – as if the body has a deeper intelligence at the cellular level that says, *Okay, I've let go of this*. Or, *Now I'm transforming the spine so I can stand straighter and also feel more emotionally stable*.

Teaching yoga is my calling

I'd describe teaching yoga as a bit like conducting a moving meditation. And it is immensely enjoyable because you're giving something of value to others. For me it's not a job, but more a state of being or 'purpose' in life. Teaching has never been about financial rewards. I remember someone once saying to me, 'Anita, what you're doing is not a real job, it's a vocation'.

'But it's very real to me,' I replied. 'Why does everything have to be measured by money alone?'

Of course, earning money is important because you need to eat and have a roof over your head, so I had to acquire a business mind over the years. But the impetus to teach was never about taking more classes to make more money – at least for me it didn't work that way. If I could live my life over again, and even if I had *heaps* of money, I would still choose the path of teaching and working with people one-to-one. I'll be 68 soon, and for as long as I can I'll continue to share yoga and meditation with others. To not share would be analogous to receiving the most extraordinary birthday present and then being told, 'You can't tell anyone about this; you have to keep this beautiful present a secret.' But how could you keep your gift a secret? You'd *have* to show everyone!

Practising yoga builds resilience and helps in coping with life, and when I refer to yoga, I mean meditation too, because meditation is an arm of yoga. Deep down, there's a knowledge that everything is part of the karmic cycle of life. I'm not saying that whatever happens in the outside world doesn't affect me, because emotionally it does, but there is an awareness that the life we view as human beings is only a tiny aspect of the whole picture. So sometimes – especially when we can't change things – it's a matter of accepting circumstances as they are.

I believe that the need to do a lot of physical yoga lessens as we age. It's not laziness, but more a matter of realising that after many years of practising meditation and yoga, you no longer need an hour of yoga practice to get into a calm state. However, this reflects my own personal experience, where I was able to reach inner stillness through starting with meditation. Others may need to practise yoga first, to calm the physical body, before being ready to sit for meditation. Of course, even though my own practice time is less these days, yoga will always be with me as a way to move, stretch and keep my body mobile. One analogy is that you can't leave your car in the garage and expect it to stay shiny and wonderful without keeping up its maintenance – because after a while it may not start! It's the same with the body.

So, as I age, my yoga practice is more about looking after my body, whereas meditation is what takes me deeper and deeper into stillness. And the great beauty of yoga is that it doesn't just move my body into poses – it steers my life in different and more fruitful directions.

The challenges of becoming vegetarian

I became a vegetarian because of my poor health – my digestion was never very strong. I remember many years ago (pre-yoga and meditation days), going to a naturopath who gave me an iridology test, and then said to me, 'Gosh, your gut! You process everything through the gut – your thoughts *and* emotions.' I was astonished to hear this.

During my Integral Yoga training, the teachers had discussed vegetarianism at length. I'd always had a reasonable diet during my life but was finding that I just couldn't digest meat any more. So, I thought about becoming a vegetarian, and started to adopt it gradually. First of all, I gave up red meat and wanted to make it clear to my family that I was serious about my dietary decision. At that time, my two boys had left home, and one was engaged. I invited the three of them to dinner one evening and cooked a roast, because they loved my roasts. When I served the meal I said, 'Okay, I'm making an announcement.' My sons already thought I was getting a bit wacky with my meditation and yoga, but they had noticed over time how happy and relaxed I'd become, and were clearly supportive.

I continued, 'This is the *last* piece of meat I will eat. I will never cook – no – I will never *eat* meat again.'

One of my sons replied, 'Oh, come on!'

'No, this is it,' I said, 'I'm never going to eat meat again; I'm becoming a vegetarian.'

My son responded, 'Oh sure, we'll see how long this lasts.'

Well, I never touched red meat again after that dinner. Initially, I still ate poultry and fish but after two years I gave up poultry and only ate fish for a while. By then I had started the Dru Yoga course, and was being introduced to ways of clearing and cleansing my body, and growing stronger energetically through the advice of several inspiring mentors (including Chris Barrington[20]). So, I took their teachings on board and also stopped eating fish, thus becoming completely vegetarian.

To my delight, I also discovered that vegetarianism isn't just about eating a few bits of lettuce and carrots. I researched the topic further and experimented with eating a variety of foods, noticing how I felt afterwards; more easily identifying the foods that were good, or not so good, for me.

Vegetarianism wasn't an ethical decision for me; it was really about gaining strength in my body and aiding digestion. As I moved deeper into yoga, meditation and vegetarianism, I gradually started to develop an ethical view about animals and how they're treated. Living in the country and being vegetarian was difficult because the locals were stock farmers, and they thought I was weird. At that time, my husband worked for a mining company which organised a Christmas function with lamb and beef on the spit, along with roast vegetables. We lined up to get our meals and the vegetables were served first. The meat was right at the end of the table with a man carving it. I was given one teeny carrot, a small potato and a few greens. I said to the girl who was serving, 'Excuse me, could I possibly have more vegetables? I'm a vegetarian and won't be eating any of the meat.'

This little lass, who must have been about 16, just looked at me. Her mouth fell open and she replied, 'That's all you're getting for now. If you don't eat meat, that's your choice. You can come back later for more vegetables, if there's any left.'

My husband said, 'Anita, don't worry, you can have mine.'

I attended several events where I went hungry, because back in those days in the country they really had no concept of vegetarianism. I was constantly trying to explain I could have vegetables but did not want meat. And I'd be told, 'But we don't serve meals that way'.

I think the worst thing that happened to me regarding vegetarianism was when I was invited to a barbecue while on holidays. I did inform the organisers in advance that I was a vegetarian, and they seemed fine with it. But when I sat down to eat, a huge plate of charred pigeons was set down right in front of me. Everyone at the barbecue was commenting, 'Isn't this great? I love the crunch of their bones!'

Out of sheer politeness I stayed, but I felt sick and couldn't bring myself to eat even my vegetarian serving. The people there had no idea I was feeling that way and my reaction surprised me too, because yoga and meditation change you from the inside out. At first you don't realise that the cells of your body are changing – and your body is becoming quite different from what it was when you first started your yoga journey. Your thinking improves too: yoga and meditation alter the way your brain works, the way you plan and how you think about life, and how you develop compassion towards others.

My life has changed so much for the better since I started practising meditation and yoga all those years ago.

REFLECTIONS

As I drove away from Anita's house, I thought about how difficult it can be sometimes to sit and connect with that quiet, still space within. At first, for many people, stiffness in the body makes sitting in meditation uncomfortable. With time and practice, yoga helps to address this through stretching the body and calming the mind. And there are numerous styles of yoga to choose from to suit different body types and needs. Most of the teachers in this book experimented with different styles before finding one that suited them best. Some people prefer a combination of gentle *asanas* (postures) and meditative practice. Others favour a strong, physical, *asana*-based practice. As Anita said, the gentle Dru Yoga that she teaches resembles a moving meditation, specialising in calming the mind and relaxing the body. At the end of class, the yoga flows effortlessly into savasana – the healing meditative rest hovering in the realm between sleep and wakefulness.

In the end it doesn't matter how we get to a point of stillness, because it's about finding what works for each of us. As we do the practices, session by session they gradually cut the mental chatter and layer by layer inner noise slows, leading to inner stillness.

Echoing what Anita said about the practices being transformative, Erich Schiffmann in his beautiful book 'Yoga the Spirit and Practice of Moving into Stillness', says:

'When you experience the peace within you, you will spontaneously undergo a fundamental transformation in the way you think about yourself and how you see the world. Nothing will seem quite the same ever again.'[21]

#5
SUSAN GRBIC

GROWING YOUNGER THROUGH YOGA

Yoga is really about finding someone inside who becomes
more and more conscious, awake, happy and connected
with the present moment

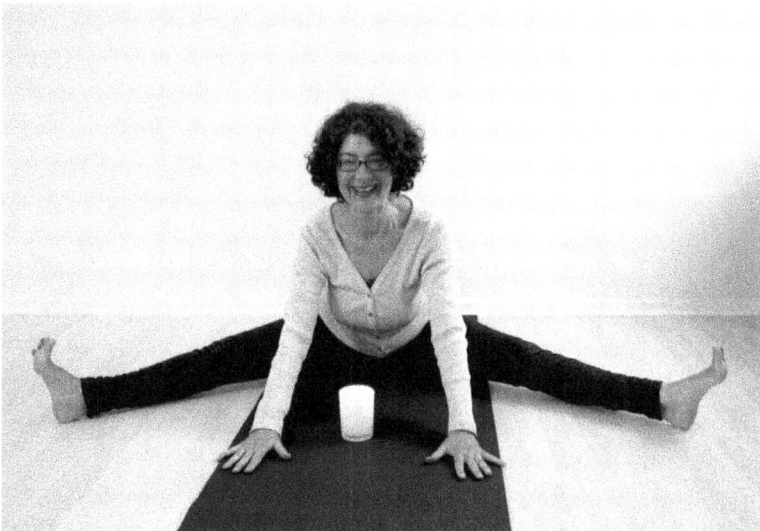

Susan in seated wide angle pose (upavishta konasana)

Yoga
With Susan
Is on Waiheke.
Hands on hearts, breathe in, breathe out
Four-part breath with flow,
Feel rested
And calm!

Susan lives on Waiheke Island (New Zealand) – a truly enchanting place, easily reached via a 40-minute ferry ride from Auckland. Before moving to Waiheke in 2012, Susan had a studio in Auckland, called the Albany Yoga Room. She has practised yoga for half her lifetime and now teaches private sessions on Waiheke in her little home studio, along with group classes in a lovely community hall nestled amongst leafy trees.

I attended Susan's Sunday morning class, which introduced me to something new: a wonderful flowing four-part breath practice, which I would like to share, as follows:

Susan's Four-Part Breath Practice

- Stand in mountain pose, straight and tall, with your arms resting down alongside the body.

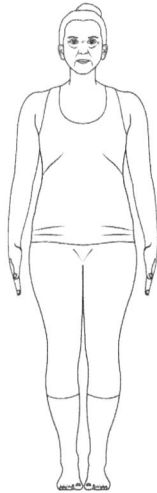

- Breathing in, raise your arms to shoulder height.

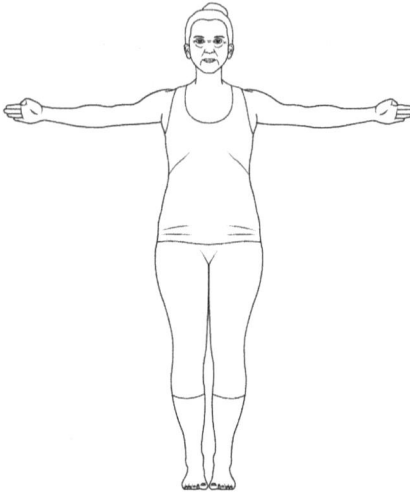

- Breathing out, bring your palms together in front of the heart.

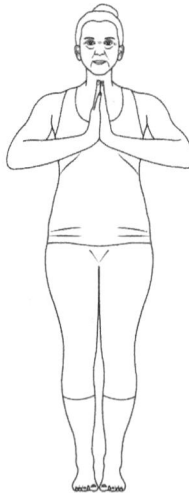

- Breathing in, straighten your arms forward, then raise them upwards in front of the head.

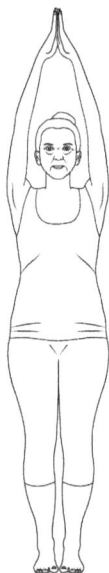

- Breathing out, take your arms out to the sides, floating them down alongside the body.

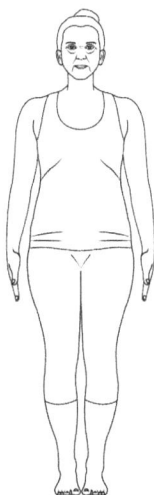

Susan took the class through a graceful, flowing sequence, using the above four-part breath, in standing forward bends and yoga lunges. It was followed by a restful, restorative pose, lying down with a bolster under the upper back to open the chest.

Susan is clearly a compassionate and experienced teacher, and she was gentle and encouraging in her instructions to: 'Explore the body and mind as if you are in a foreign country.' And so I did, and by the end of the class I felt totally relaxed and peaceful.

After class, we held our interview sitting on a comfy lounge in a tearoom adjacent to the hall. Susan offers a thought-provoking perspective on ageing: what she describes as 'adhering to the principles of growing younger'; taking a different view to the common societal focus on what we 'lose' as we age – instead, focusing on what we 'gain'. Here's the story of how Susan's experiences with yoga (and interconnected practices) guided her to this heartening point of view.

SUSAN'S STORY

My yoga journey begins

My journey towards yoga started in 1977 through discovering Transcendental Meditation (TM).[22] In those days, I was an air hostess with South African Airways, which was a stressful and erratic lifestyle. Flying causes the body's systems to become unbalanced, and because you're constantly moving into different time zones, everything feels back to front. I worked as an air hostess for just over three years and during that time I started practising TM for stress release. One day, on a first-class flight to London, I found myself working alongside a steward whom I'd never met before. We started talking about meditation and one of the points he made deeply resonated with me: 'All meditation is good,' he said, 'and TM is fine, but do understand that TM is just a mental exercise; it's never going to take you beyond the realm of the mind – it's not a *true* spiritual practice.'

At first, I had no idea what he was talking about but I soon discovered what he meant. I had become a vegetarian by then, and on my next flight I was sitting in the galley eating a fruit salad. One of the stewards came in and said, 'Oh, that looks nice.' He was also a vegetarian, and sat down with me to eat his fruit salad. We started talking and I found out he was on the same spiritual path as the steward I'd met the previous week. Our flight was going to Mauritius and by the time we'd finished the trip, which included two days of relaxing on a beach, this steward had told me all about 'the spiritual path'. I realised it was what I'd been looking for all my life – and was terrified that I might be run over by a bus before I became initiated! But nothing awful happened and I'm still here. I was initiated into Sant Mat[23], in Johannesburg, and subsequently travelled to India to spend time with my spiritual Master, Maharaj Charan Singh. You know the old adage: *When the pupil is ready, the master appears.* I didn't find him – he found me through those two airline stewards – and I've continued on this particular spiritual path since 1980.

I became involved in yoga in 1985, when I was living in Cape Town, South Africa. I was pregnant for the first time and felt that

I really needed to learn how to breathe correctly. So, I went along to ante-natal yoga classes and thoroughly enjoyed them. I don't know which style of yoga I was practising then, but it was gentle.

After I gave birth to my first daughter, a friend took me along to an Iyengar Yoga[24] class. I initially found the practices very hard on my body and didn't want to continue the classes. However, my friend dragged me back for a second class and from then on, I was hooked!

I continued with Iyengar Yoga, but in 1993 decided to sign up for a one-year teacher training course with a different style of yoga, called Integral Yoga.[25] Compared with Iyengar, Integral Yoga is not so strongly focused on physical *asana*: it moves more towards meditation, breathing practices and yogic philosophy. So, through my teacher training studies with Integral Yoga, I discovered the 'other side' of yoga and went on to complete my teacher training exams early (as my family and I had decided to emigrate to New Zealand before the year was up).

Settling in New Zealand with my husband, three small daughters and elderly mother – after our huge move half way across the world – I really needed to find some yoga classes! Although I was now a qualified Integral Yoga teacher, I hadn't yet started teaching, so I decided to attend Iyengar classes as a student again. However, in 1996, when my youngest daughter began school, I felt strongly that I wanted to start teaching yoga, so I talked to my Iyengar teacher, Joy, about the possibility. She agreed, knowing how dedicated I was but advised me that to qualify I'd first have to complete an Iyengar teacher training intensive.

So, I completed a 10-day intensive training with Felicity

Green, a prominent American Iyengar teacher who was visiting New Zealand at that time. I then taught my very first class at Joy's studio, North Shore Yoga, in Auckland. Following this, Joy kindly offered me her Iyengar teacher training course for free, as I was to be her first trainee! In all, I completed two years of teacher training with Joy, as well as assisting in all her classes and learning the poses and adjustments required for the final teaching assessment. This was over 20 years ago, and at that time there weren't as many strict rules as there are now regarding Iyengar teacher training requirements.

When I finally applied for my official Iyengar teaching assessment, I was nervous and keen to get it over and done with. In those days, there were no qualified assessors in New Zealand; they had to come from Australia. I was stunned and disappointed when the Iyengar assessors informed me that they wouldn't be coming to New Zealand, as there weren't enough trainees that year to warrant assessment. The following year I was notified that assessments would be conducted (as there were enough trainees), but to be honest, I was so over it all by then that I told the assessors I was no longer interested in receiving a teaching certificate. So, although I'd completed all the necessary training and the required hours on the mat, I never received a teaching qualification. To this day, I don't call myself an Iyengar teacher, although I am allowed to say that my classes are Iyengar-based.

Adjustments, injuries and other important lessons

When I first started teaching, one of the most valuable lessons was that my adjustments[26] had to be both *present* and *conscious*. In those early days, I remember placing my hand on a student's thigh and pressing down, perhaps more forcibly than required. The student didn't say anything at the time, but I sensed I shouldn't have done this, as that student never returned to my classes. Today, when I teach a private one-on-one class, I advise my student: 'During our session, I will correct your pose with hands-on adjustments, but if you don't want to be touched tell me now. And during an adjustment, you need to tell me if the pressure is too firm for you, as each person's body is different.'

I suffered an injury in 2007, fracturing my sternum while I was showing an advanced class how to place their hands on a partner in the downward-facing dog pose (in order to give a stronger hamstring stretch). In the downward-facing dog pose, it's often difficult for people to press their heels to the floor without force, so I advised the class to have their heels propped up against the wall, or to roll a blanket and place it under both heels, for support and grounding.

To demonstrate this adjustment for the class, one student agreed to be my partner, but while I was speaking to the group, I hadn't noticed that she'd placed a blanket flat under her feet, instead of rolling it up under her heels. As I leaned towards her and gently pushed, she was not secured and her feet slipped. We both went for a tumble, and I was accidentally thumped in the breastbone. For a moment, I was winded and couldn't speak; my students were concerned, but I assured them I was fine and continued with the class.

I was in pain after class but thought it might just be due to bruising. I visited a chiropractor who told me there appeared to be a small hairline fracture in the sternum, and two ribs were dislocated. To give my body time to heal, I didn't work for a few weeks, and just wandered around at home – which was rather nice! Fortunately, I knew several wonderful teachers who were able to cover my classes. During that period of recovery, my meditation and yoga practices included a 'healing visualisation' in the injured parts of my body, and I practised deep relaxation. A friend also gave me a wholistic therapy called Body Talk, which is believed to stimulate the body's innate ability to balance and *heal* itself. In retrospect, I feel that the combination of all these practices helped me to recover.

Another big lesson for me when I was a new teacher was learning how to pace a class. On one occasion, at short notice, I was asked to teach the Tuesday morning class on behalf of my teacher, Joy. By this time, I'd been attending her classes for several years and was well acquainted with the other students. Now suddenly, I was switching roles from fellow student to their teacher! Well, I planned that class down to the very last breath, but ended up not fitting all the practices in. Afterwards, one of my fellow students gave me the feedback that it was enjoyable, but a bit too slow.

Of course, initially when you start teaching, it's important to prepare classes methodically. Now, as an experienced teacher, I often *ad lib*: there's a vague class plan in my head but then I make it up as I go along, because every class should cater to the needs of each student present on that specific day.

I'm also conscious that sometimes I talk too much when I'm teaching; however, it's the 'Iyengar way' to teach with an abundance of instructions, to ensure that students practise the poses correctly. However, I personally feel that most students don't need more than about three instructions for a pose; the teacher must allow some 'quiet time' so that students can connect with feelings and sensations as they arise and find their own inner balance and alignment. One of the key challenges for teachers is finding this balance between giving instructions and allowing students to explore the poses for themselves.

So, all these experiences have helped me to understand that teaching yoga is about balancing the following aspects:

- managing hands-on adjustments with care and awareness;
- pacing from one pose to the next (how fast or slow);
- gauging how many instructions to give;
- learning when to talk and when to be quiet; and
- with injury, knowing when to stop and rest so the body can recover.

New directions with Iyengar Yoga

After teaching at North Shore Yoga for about five years, I decided to open my own studio in partnership with another established Iyengar teacher, Stephanie, and in 2000 we opened Albany Yoga Room. During our first year in the studio, we attended a workshop in Tauranga, run by Donna Farhi[27] (one of the first workshops she held in New Zealand). Until I'd met Donna, I was strictly Iyengar based and was truly astounded when during the workshop she said, 'Just be a bit creative, this is *your* practice; be free with it and make it your own.'

In 15 years of practising Iyengar Yoga no one had ever given me permission to be myself. Of course, I'm grateful for my earlier Iyengar grounding, because I believe there is no better way to start off in yoga, and to teach it, than having Iyengar as a foundation. Anyway, I found Donna just amazing; I invited her to present a weekend workshop at Albany Yoga Room the following year, and from then on I hosted her workshops annually. Over time, the weekend workshops extended into five-day intensives. I worked with Donna numerous times, and often travelled down to the South Island for her women's yoga retreats. She completely radicalised my whole way of thinking about yoga, and how I practise and teach it to this day. Physical *asana* practice is an important vehicle, but for me it's not the sole purpose of yoga and hasn't been for a long time. For so many years, despite my spiritual leanings and interest in meditation, my yoga practice was still very much *asana*-based until I met Donna. From then on, my practice started evolving into something much softer, with a more fluid approach. Donna was undoubtedly my true mentor.

Politics in the yoga world

When I first started practising Iyengar Yoga in the mid-1980s, every other style of yoga was what my first Iyengar teacher called 'fruit salad yoga' – a little bit of everything, all mixed together. Until Iyengar Yoga came along, there was limited understanding of the intricacies of *asanas*. Unless the teachers were very well trained, the way poses were taught was sometimes sloppy, careless and even unsafe. Then Iyengar became 'the way to go' and, as devotees of this style, we thought our yoga was superior. When Ashtanga Yoga[28] became a popular school of yoga, several Iyengar people rolled their eyes because they felt that Ashtanga teachers didn't explain how to perform *asanas* properly. The Ashtanga teachers themselves held the view that teaching yoga was about working with the breath and movement. Yoga became further politicised as other styles, including Bikram Yoga[29] emerged on the global scene. Popular yoga became increasingly focused on making the practices harder, raising a sweat, losing weight and getting a strong workout.

I tried a Bikram Yoga class once, where we practised a range of difficult standing poses, one after the other in a room heated somewhere between 35–42 degrees celsius. Halfway through the class I felt like I was going to be sick, so I moved to leave the room.

The teacher said to me, 'You can't leave the class.'

'I have to get out,' I said.

'No,' she replied. 'Lie down on the floor.'

I ignored her, walking out of the class into the change room where it was cool. I lay down on the floor and rested with my legs up on the bench, until I felt better. Afterwards I realised I'd been in the men's change room! I returned to finish the class, but it was just revolting; the guy next to me was drenched in sweat which kept splattering onto my mat. The weird thing was that I actually felt good after the class, but I was adamant, *I don't care how good I feel, I'm never going back!*

If you're planning to practise Bikram or Power Yoga or something similar, these styles will make you strong and fit, but they might not introduce you to the 'real' yoga journey. Donna Farhi once told me that she was waiting at a reception area in a yoga studio in North America, and overheard people asking, 'How much of a workout do we get here?' That was their only interest. Personally, I feel the 'workout' attitude gave rise to teachers like us questioning yoga's direction in our culture and introducing a whole new way of thinking about it, including: integrating the breathing practices, spiritual aspects and internal connection – and diminishing the obsession with just the physical aspects.

The tree of yoga has so many different branches. Unfortunately, in the West, the popular part of yoga (about 90 percent) is all about the physical body: the execution of beautiful *asanas* and wearing trendy yoga gear. In my view, this completely misses the point of what yoga is truly about, which is 'connecting us to our source'. My daughters are apt at reminding me, 'Don't worry Ma, because remember that's where *you* started yoga as well, thinking all about the body.' So, I've accepted that with some people, physical yoga will lead them to something deeper, whereas with others it won't.

I'm also concerned that without a wholistic focus people can injure themselves through practising yoga. In New Zealand, we have an accidental injury compensation scheme (ACC), which insures the whole population. As a self-employed yoga teacher, I'm required to pay into ACC. There are different categories depending on how difficult or dangerous your activity is ranked, and yoga is categorised as a sport, because so many people are injured through its practice.

Growing younger with yoga

When I moved to Waiheke Island in 2012, I started to think about what it meant to grow older, and for a while I explored the idea of 'growing younger' which included looking at what we can *gain* through ageing – at an emotional, mental and spiritual level – rather than focusing negatively on things we *lose* or leave behind. From my own practices and study over many years, I've learnt that a combination of yoga, meditation, mindfulness, healthy living habits and the practice of virtues (such as kindness, compassion and gratitude), all have profound beneficial effects on the individual, and those around us.

While I'm not as physically fit as when I was younger, I'm still as agile and healthy, and in fact, I feel like a teenager around 80 percent of the time! Occasionally my body does feel oddly different, as if I'm inhabiting a foreign being – one that's painful, tired, old or stiff. Friends often grumble about getting old, but most of the time I don't feel a day older than on my wedding day all those years ago – and that's a key benefit of yoga.

Looking at my own health needs as I age, the yoga pose I practise most is a supported backbend, lying over a bolster placed under the upper back to open my chest.

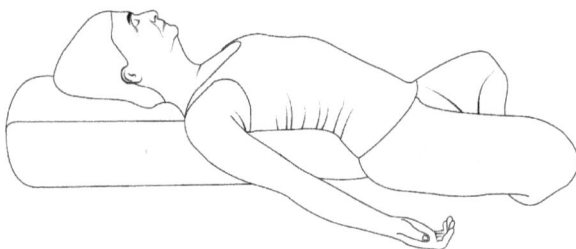

My mother had inherited severe kyphosis, a rounding of the spine. I was also very rounded in the upper back when I first started yoga, so I started lying over a bolster every day at the beginning of my practice and it radically changed my skeletal structure. I can honestly say that my spine has straightened out substantially. My daughters inherited kyphosis as well, but since starting yoga, their spines look a lot better. My favourite pose though is *viparita karani*; the restorative pose with a bolster under my pelvis and legs stretched up the wall. It's so relaxing!

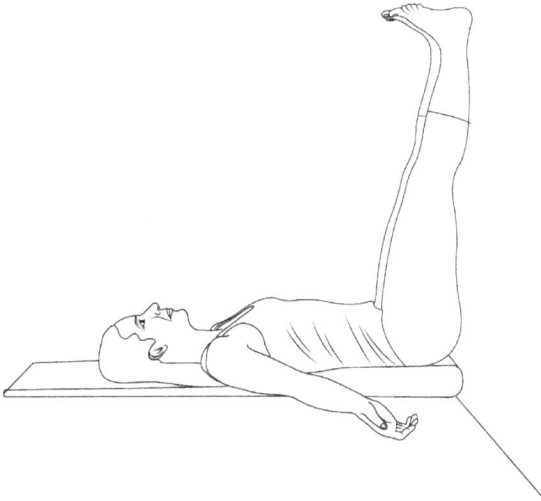

Cultivating finer qualities and feelings through yoga

Practising yoga also helps to cultivate higher qualities and values, and one of the most important is the ability to feel gratitude. More than anything, I want my students to understand this aspect of yoga and work towards nurturing these feelings, rather than just stretching their hamstrings. I believe yoga is really about finding 'someone inside' who becomes more and more conscious, awake, happy and connected with the present moment. Many women start my classes in their fifties and sixties and they love it! As newcomers, they often walk up the stairs to the studio looking anxious and tense, but after class they leave looking radiant, smiling and happy – and they start to carry this light-hearted quality with them throughout the day.

Self-compassion is another important quality that yoga helps to develop. When I was running the Albany Yoga Room in Auckland it was hectic: I taught eight yoga classes a week, whilst running the business and taking care of a husband and three young children – so when I could, I cut down to six classes a week. These days, I call myself semi-retired: I teach two classes a week, and on average do three private one-on-one classes. As I've aged, my physical practice has also softened; I'm much kinder to myself these days. And getting out of bed on cold Waiheke mornings to do my early morning practice is sometimes challenging!

I practise meditation virtually every day for about half an hour, and yoga on most days for half an hour or longer, depending on how I feel. I still perform headstands and shoulder stands, but my practice is not as vigorous as before, it's become more breath-directed and internalised. I also feel less pressured because I don't have to be like a 25-year-old anymore. Well, I'm nearly 67 after all! And as I grow older, I also realise that *I'm* the boss regarding my yoga practice – it's up to me whether I enjoy it or beat myself up about it – and I choose to make it enjoyable. Self-compassion has taught me to respect my body as I age, because it doesn't bounce back quite as quickly.

Yoga and meditation have been my constant companions through all the 'ups and downs' of life; they remain my guiding stars, giving me direction whenever I need it. Looking back, if I had discovered only my spiritual path (and this includes meditation but not hatha yoga), I think my life would have turned out quite differently. If I hadn't found *either* of these paths, I can't imagine how I would have coped in life, because when I look at the world, I see it's completely mad and getting madder all the time. Without the bigger picture that yoga has given me, the world would appear to be *hell*. I want to say to everyone, 'Just understand that everything is actually perfect – as awful as these terrible things happening in the world can seem to us – we only perceive such a tiny piece of this so-called "reality".'

Another way of thinking about life, which yoga has helped me develop, is that we are all part of nature, and as everything in nature evolves perfectly, so do we. The problem is that we keep getting in our own way, trying to stop life's natural flow or change its course, which we can't. Perhaps we just need to learn to 'go with it' – like a tree, blossoming and dropping its leaves at the right time, and not trying to control nature's processes.

Without a doubt, practising yoga has made me happier, more patient, tolerant and conscious. When I was younger, I was cynical, but now all of that cynicism has vanished. The older I grow, the happier I am, and life is becoming even more exciting and enjoyable – little things make me feel contented now. Yoga has attained that for me. Today, looking around at Waiheke, this island paradise, I wonder how I came to be living in such a beautiful place. And rather than putting it purely down to luck, I do increasingly believe that one's thinking creates intention and reality in life.

My sincere wish is for everyone to find the right yoga and meditation practice to help them feel happy, healthy and at ease with life. I do think it's such a pity if a person tries one or two yoga classes, doesn't have a good experience and just gives up. Please believe me when I say there is always a teacher and style of yoga out there that will suit you.

RELECTIONS

After we finished the interview, Susan hurried off to have some 'mum and daughter time' with one of her daughters who was visiting from the mainland. I wandered down to the local village of Oneroa, pondering Susan's ideas about ageing. As Susan described to me: meditation, yoga and other mindfulness practices, enable a different kind of consciousness to emerge about life and ageing – and this has been fundamental to her happiness. She has rejected limiting stereotypical mindsets around ageing, because for her they just don't fit – she's remade ageing to her own specifications; it has become an exciting time of change, wisdom and transformation, with much to be gained, and opportunities to learn more about one's 'self'.

If all this seems a little far-fetched then consider the studies about mindful ageing by the famous American, Harvard University Professor, Ellen Langer. Langer argues that what you think and do at any age can make a difference to your quality of life and health. In her famous 'Counter Clockwise' study, in 1979, she took a group of elderly men to a timeless retreat, for one week, where they lived as if it was 1959 (20 years earlier than it was). The men were requested to refer to their families and careers as if they were back in 1959, and all the paraphernalia was set up to represent that time period. Basically, they were required to act as if they were 20 years younger, and still aged in their late fifties and early sixties. The men appeared to grow younger: their bodies showed improvement in physical strength, perception, cognition, taste, hearing and visual thresholds. Langer states: 'Over time I have come to believe less and less that biology is destiny. It is not primarily our physical selves that limit us but rather our mindset about our physical limits.'[30]

When we look around at all the stereotypical portrayals of ageing, in the media and elsewhere, it seems hardly surprising that most people view ageing with trepidation, and as a time of loss and decline. Yet it doesn't have to be this way. Joseph F. Coughlin (Director of the Massachusetts Institute of Technology Age Lab) calls widespread negative notions about ageing, which categorise older people as one uniform group, 'a mass delusion'.[31]

So how can we free ourselves from constricting mindsets and the limits they place on our health and wellbeing as we age? Just as Langer argues, through practising mindful ageing with present moment awareness (focusing on what is happening right here, right now, not thinking about the past or worrying about the future), actively seeking new experiences, and accepting that we can and do change – the self-same pathway along which yoga and meditation and other mindfulness practices lead us. And Susan's beautiful knowing smile, in her photo at the start of the chapter, says it all.

#6
BETTE CALMAN

RELAX, RESET AND RECHARGE THE BODY

Yoga grants no immunity from life's inevitable fluxes and trials,
but its practice cultivates resilience, calmness and acceptance

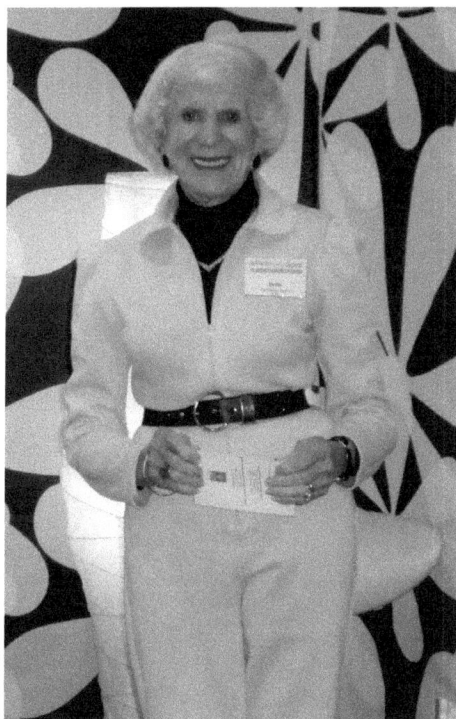

Bette Calman in a 'cat suit'

Meet Bette
At 91.
Many memories.
Teacher for some 60 years,
TV yoga star
In cat suits
Doyenne!

In 2011, Guinness World Records listed Bette Calman (then aged 85) as the world's oldest female yoga teacher — she had been teaching yoga for nearly 60 years. Now retired, Bette still practises yoga.

As a child in the 1960s, I loved watching Bette demonstrate yoga on Jaye Walton's popular Adelaide-based, day-time television show, A Touch of Elegance. Bette was awe-inspiring, twisting her body into bendy postures with glamour and ease. She's also renowned for her stunning collection of catsuits. If you're wondering what a catsuit is, it's the 1980s equivalent of the onesie (jumpsuit), but tight-fitting and made from stretchy material. Bette always wore hers with a belt around the waist (see opening page photo). She designed these suits herself, sketching them up, then engaging a dressmaker to make the garments.

Two days before our scheduled interview, Bette had an unexpected hospital admission and her daughter, Susie, contacted me. I suggested we postpone the meeting, but Susie assured me that Bette was still looking forward to seeing me and talking about yoga. Susie knew I was coming by train, so we decided to meet at her house, which is close to Williamstown Station in Melbourne. On the morning of our meeting, as I sat on a train travelling across the city, it was with mixed feelings: excitement and nervousness tinged with curiosity. I wondered what Bette would be like: it was 20 years or more since I had last seen her. She was my very first yoga teacher back in the 1990s (in Adelaide), and introduced me to the wonders of yoga in an old, draughty church hall.

I found Bette exactly as I remembered her: still petite, and exuding radiant calm energy and vitality – a testament to the benefits of her lifelong yoga practice. She told me that one of her favourite books is Yoga for Women[32], which is also a popular book with many of the other contributors to Yoga Years. Yoga for Women is very much a product of its time (the 1960s), promising women 'poise', 'magnetism', 'joy in living' and a 'slim figure', if yoga is practised regularly. Nevertheless, observing Bette, all these claims seemed true.

I asked Bette to let me know if she felt tired during our interview or wanted to take a break at any time. Her heartfelt response was, 'I could talk about yoga all day long'. Bette is a passionate advocate for the benefits of yoga to health and wellbeing. What follows is the story of her incredible yoga journey.

BETTE'S STORY

Yearning for yoga

I yearned to try yoga from my early teens, but numerous obstacles stood in the way, and many years would pass by before I could fulfil my longing. When I was about 15, the English 'yoga guru' Sir Paul Dukes[33] visited Sydney. This was in the 1940s, going back nearly 80 years now, and yoga was not as widely accepted then as it is today. My mother thought yoga was very strange and didn't understand why people wanted to stand on their heads. My father was more philosophical, so I hoped he might let me attend Sir Paul's classes. We sat down together to talk about it, and he asked me, 'Why do you want to go?'

I replied, 'I don't know Dad, I just want to.'

Unfortunately, that wasn't a good enough reason, so I wasn't given permission to attend Sir Paul's classes.

During the 1940s, I wanted to learn more about yoga, but just couldn't find any relevant books to guide me. In fact, I had to wait another decade until Angus and Robertson (the main book store in Sydney) obtained copies of *Yoga and Health* (1953) by Selvarajan Yesudian and Elisabeth Haich.[34] I still find it an incredibly beautiful and sensibly written book. I also remember attending a talk that Yesudian gave about yoga when he visited Australia. English was his second language, but he explained yoga as clearly as he could; it made a lot of sense and yoga sounded like the perfect practice for me.

Anyway, it wasn't until I was in my late twenties that I finally attended a yoga class. The Michael Volin Yoga School[35] had opened in Sydney in 1950, and I experienced my first class there. I loved it from the start and became a regular student. However, it would be over a decade more before I eventually became a yoga teacher. I started my teacher training with Michael, when he invited me to accompany him to classes at Double Bay, so that I could observe his style of instruction. I was thrilled when he selected me to train as a teacher. My yoga teacher training was taught orally (a more traditional way of training) and I was also required to attend classes with Michael for several more years.

One day, Michael told me he was planning to set up new yoga classes in North Bondi, and he invited me to teach them. So, off I went to teach my very first class – but no-one turned up! Perhaps the students realised it would just be me, a brand-new teacher, taking the class. But deep down I felt self-assured that I was meant to teach, despite having small numbers of students in my classes for quite some time.

Teaching yoga in a pub lounge

My yoga classes were finally becoming established in Sydney when I moved to Adelaide (with my husband Bruce) to manage a new pub, the Hotel Enfield. In those days, yoga was virtually unheard of in Adelaide: as far as I knew, the only two names associated there with yoga were Iris Clutterham and Ian Burey.[36] So, when I started teaching yoga in the hotel lounge, my classes filled an empty niche: the students started to come and just kept on coming! Although it was a lovely lounge, a hotel was not an ideal place to teach yoga. We were also living on-site, and I was supposed to be working in the hotel with Bruce.

Bruce and I were married for 58 years. He didn't practise yoga, but found the relaxations beneficial for the various illnesses he suffered from over the years. Of course, yoga was the perfect activity for me, keeping me healthy and providing the energy I needed to work long hours in the hotel. Yoga was also an antidote for relieving my tired, aching legs from standing up all day. At the end of a long day, I would close the bedroom door and go 'upside-down' into a headstand to give my legs a much-needed rest.

Opening the Bette Calman Yoga School

After I'd been living in Adelaide for a few years, Michael Volin suggested that I open a yoga school there, and he added, 'I'll send Nancy Phelan down to help you.' Nancy was Michael's assistant teacher in Sydney, and together they co-wrote 14 books on yoga, including *Yoga for Women*. Unfortunately, just before Nancy was due to travel to Adelaide, she broke her arm and had to cancel the trip. Consequently, I opened the yoga school myself. I found a hall at 16 Waymouth Street (in the Adelaide CBD) and organised its refurbishment, making it a comfy place for classes. The Bette Calman Yoga School was popular from the start and I was soon putting on extra classes. There was a six o'clock class scheduled almost every evening and the constant demand for classes never ceased. I worked very hard teaching, but it was always enjoyable. After some time, I started training suitable students to become yoga teachers, and we held classes in the suburbs for the trainees who couldn't travel to the city studio. In those days, teacher training consisted of meeting with the trainees once a week, where they would come along and observe a yoga class as a way of learning new poses. After class, we would discuss each session in detail, and the trainees would then prepare their lesson plans based on these collective experiences.

My yoga classes grew very large, and once I taught a class at the Masonic Hall in Adelaide to over 250 students. I also supplied all the mats: each student was given two green yoga mats made from foam carpet padding (this was before modern 'sticky' mats were invented). I remember on that day, with such a large group there were nowhere near enough mats to go around! It's still hard to believe, but there I was, up on the stage, teaching so many people. I had never seen so many students in a class before. I recall it was exactly 254 people because one of my assistants took down all their names and addresses. But my general daily classes averaged around 20 students for each session. Students were mixed in age and gender, and came from different backgrounds, including: accountants, housewives, schoolteachers and garbage collectors.

'A Touch of Elegance'

One day I was giving a demonstration about yoga in Adelaide, and Jaye Walton (a prominent television host) was there. She approached me and said, 'I'm opening a show on television called *A Touch of Elegance* and I'd like you to do a guest presentation about yoga.' The show started in 1968 and was a mix of fashion, lifestyle segments and interviews with celebrities. I would be at the TV studio once a week, dressed in a lovely leotard and demonstrating yoga poses. I ended up doing the yoga spot for that show once a week for over 20 years; it always went well, and nothing ever felt like an effort because I loved doing it.

Then I was offered a weekly column about yoga in Adelaide's evening newspaper, and in the 1970s, Rigby (the Adelaide book publishers) approached me to write a series of small books on yoga, which I agreed to do. I selected book topics that highlighted yoga as a therapy for a range of conditions, including: *Yoga for Weight Control*, *Yoga for Arthritis,* and *Yoga for Relaxation.*[37] Writing these books became quite a workload for me, as Rigby continued to republish them and wanted new book ideas as well. I was fortunate to have Joan Brodie, my co-author, helping to produce them.

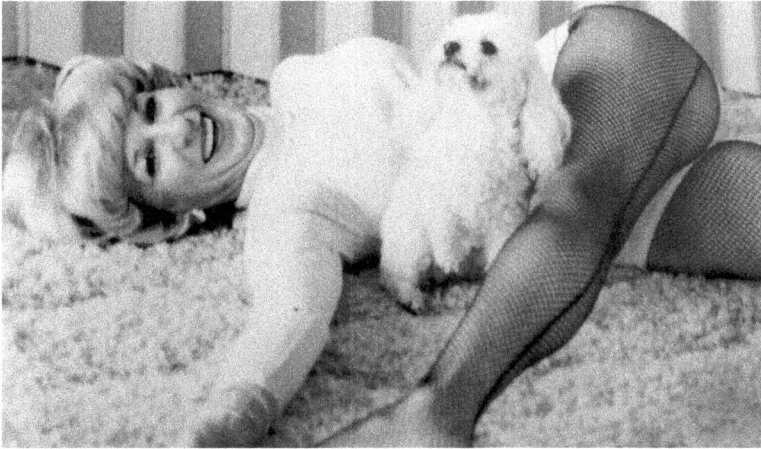

Yoga with Bette Calman and poodle (circa 1980s)
(South Australian Magazine, SAM)

In addition to the above titles, I wrote a book called *General Health Rules*, which was published through the Bette Calman Yoga Centre.

Going with the flow

By the mid-1980s, Bruce and I were well and truly settled in Adelaide, but then our daughter Susie's marriage broke up. She was living in Melbourne with two young children to care for and Bruce suggested we move there to help her with the kids. Initially I was against the idea, as I *loathed* Melbourne – in fact, we both did. I even told Susie that we wouldn't be moving there. But one night my little granddaughter, who was only about six at the time, phoned me and was crying, 'Nanna, when are you coming to Melbourne? Mummy says you're not coming.'

I found myself saying to her, 'We're coming at the end of the month.'

So, Bruce and I moved to Melbourne and settled there permanently. Looking back, although we didn't want to move, it was really the right thing to do; we were able to help Susie so much with the children. She was teaching yoga at that time, and could depend on us picking up the kids from school. I also helped Susie set up her yoga classes whenever I had time, as she would often have 30 to 40 students to prepare for in a class.

In Melbourne, I continued to teach up to 11 yoga classes each week until I was 85 and decided to retire. One place I taught at was a 'women-only' gym. Fortunately for me, the wife of the owner wouldn't let any noise penetrate from the other gym rooms while my yoga class was running. In fact, she policed it so well that my classes grew consistently until they were very large. I taught numerous students there for many years, and we bonded, becoming great friends. I still see this marvellous group of women, even though I don't teach them yoga any more. We get together for birthday lunches and other celebrations.

'Tick off' and reset your body

What I enjoyed most about teaching yoga for all those years was feeling marvellous after every single class. I never came out of a class without feeling better than before I went in. And that's how it's supposed to be! Unfortunately, I don't think this is true of all yoga classes today; the way yoga is taught has changed a lot. After attending other teachers' classes I've often wondered, *Well, what was that all about?*

I believe that to get a boost in mood you must 'tick off the body'. By this, I mean working all the way through every part of the body, following the comprehensive system Michael Volin used: bending forward; leaning backwards; bending sideways; doing a breathing technique; and having a relaxation at the start *and* end of each class. Michael's system even included sequences to exercise your eyes, for example: 'moving around the clock'. The way he balanced his classes was truly beautiful. As a student, you always knew what was coming next, although the postures varied depending on who was in class on the day, because Michael taught at the individual student's level. Even with age, my own teaching style and practice didn't really change structurally.

In my view, today there is too much emphasis on making the yoga poses look physically beautiful. I've been lucky during my lifetime, as I could perform most of the poses with ease – yoga always felt natural to me. But it's important to understand what these poses are *for*, and to realise the powerful effects they can have on the body.

In contrast, nowadays there seems to be less emphasis on breathing practices and relaxations; yet everyone is so busy, stress is endemic and these practices offer the perfect remedy. Relaxation practices allow valuable 'quiet time'; a chance to let go of thinking and bring the body into stillness. In my classes, I used to teach relaxation for 10 minutes at the beginning and end of a class. I've noticed that teachers today often only give a few minutes rest at the end of class, without any quiet time at the beginning. Michael Volin always emphasised that the first relaxation in class was very important, because it allowed students time to let go of the outside world and leave their problems behind for a while. Then having released some of the tensions, stresses and worries of everyday life they were ready to start their yoga practice. I remember some students would regularly arrive late to his classes, but Michael was strict: he wouldn't let anyone in the door halfway through the relaxation, so these latecomers would miss the relaxation entirely. I recall in my classes the students looked noticeably different after relaxations – always younger and healthier.

Yoga contributes to positive health on so many levels: poses keep the body supple through stretching and movement, and I do feel that we hold our shape better through yoga practice, even as we age. Yogis also spend quite a lot of time sitting on the floor. Have you noticed how older people, who don't practise yoga, find it difficult to get down onto and up from the floor? However, this needn't discourage the elderly from trying yoga, because they can always start by sitting in a chair.

On a deeper level, I do believe that yoga expands self-awareness and helps people to move in more positive and creative directions in life.

Thoughts on food, injuries and acceptance

I've been a vegetarian for over 40 years now, and feel that a plant-based diet is what my body needs. But just because this type of diet works for me, that doesn't mean it's right for everyone. Eat what feels good for you and don't feel guilty about it. My attitude about food is: if you want to eat a piece of cake, then *enjoy* it rather than letting the decision cause conflict in your mind –

don't waste energy criticising yourself!

Looking at my current physical health, recently I've had two falls. In the first one I injured myself quite badly when I fell over backwards and broke my wrist. I also damaged my shoulder, although this wasn't detected at the time. Later, during a massage, the masseuse asked if my shoulder was sore, as it was swollen, but I hadn't realised it was injured as there was no obvious pain. Unfortunately, that damaged shoulder has now swollen to twice the size of the other, and it creaks when I move it. Having these falls really changed me – I became frightened. Then I started to lose my eyesight: my vision suddenly went dark, like a shutter closing over a camera. I thought, *My eyesight's gone.* Fortunately, I didn't lose it, but I do have to take special care of my eyes these days.

I also have limitations with certain yoga poses. Before my first fall, I could hold one leg straight up and then out to the side for a long time, but I can't manage this anymore. However, I've noticed that you *can* keep practising yoga as you age, because if one system shuts down then another starts to open. What's important is not to push your practice too hard, and to *listen* to your body. My favourite pose used to be Salute to the Sun, but I haven't tried to do it lately, due to the fragility of my eyes. I can still get down on the floor and take my legs up to full shoulder stand and its variations, but I avoid the full plough pose (where the legs are lowered behind the head towards the floor) due to my sore shoulder. So, there are a few things I can't manage and I accept that. Of course, I can still practise relaxation and breathing exercises – they are vital, as they recharge and revitalise me.

Even now with my physical limitations, none of it bothers me. I have truly loved my life and all the things I've accomplished. I've led a charmed life and yoga has been a precious part of it, and still is. Yoga helps me 'live for today'.

REFLECTIONS

Bette and I spent a long time chatting after we'd completed the interview. Over several cups of tea, we talked about our mutual love of yoga and all its benefits for the body and mind. When we finished, I sent an SMS to Susie saying, 'I just left your place. Thanks so much for organising things with Bette.' A short time later, I received her response: 'My pleasure. Bette is in savasana, as I type.'

I stopped at a café down the road to have lunch, reflecting on Bette's insights and taking time to digest them along with the food. I remembered how several months before, as I was packing to move house, some small coloured slips of paper fell out of one of my books. The titles on them were 'A Smile' (see image below); 'Yoga – Rules of Living'; and 'A Simple Reflection'. I was given these handwritten mementoes at Bette's yoga classes in Adelaide in the 1990s. She would place them on the floor next to her students when they were in savasana (relaxation) at the end of a class. They were a wonderful keepsake to focus on until the next class.

A SMILE

+ A SMILE costs nothing, but gives much.
+ It enriches those who receive, without making poorer those who give.
+ It takes but a moment, but the memory of it sometimes lasts forever.
+ None is so rich or mighty that he can get along without it, and none is so poor, but that he can be made rich by it.
+ A SMILE creates happiness in the home, fosters good will in business, and is the countersign of friendship.
+ It brings rest to the weary, cheer to the discouraged, sunshine to the sad, and it is natures best antitode for trouble.
+ Yet it cannot be bought, begged, borrowed, or stolen, for it is something that is of no value to anyone until it is given away.
+ Some people are too tired to give you a SMILE.
+ Give them one of yours, as none needs a SMILE so much, as he who has no more to give.

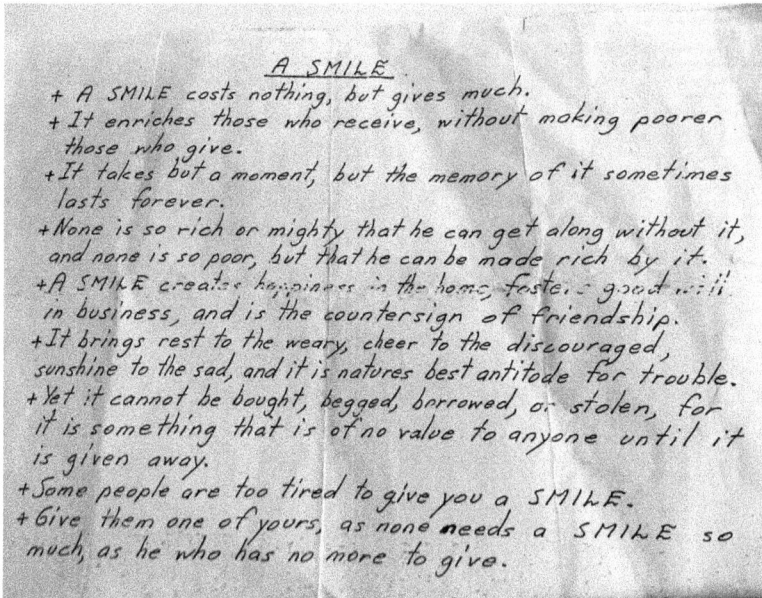

'A Smile', handout from Bette Calman's
yoga class, circa mid-1990s.

After lunch I made my way on foot to Williamstown Harbour, to catch a ferry to Southbank in the city. It was a lovely, calm journey on the water, much like the interview with Bette and the practice of yoga itself. Yoga grants no immunity from life's inevitable fluxes and trials, but as Bette demonstrates, its practice cultivates resilience, calmness and acceptance – with a focus on the present moment, and positive aspects of life.

#7
SHEILA HAYES

SAFE YOGA FOR SENIORS

Yoga has been my life journey – and I've never regretted
a single moment of it

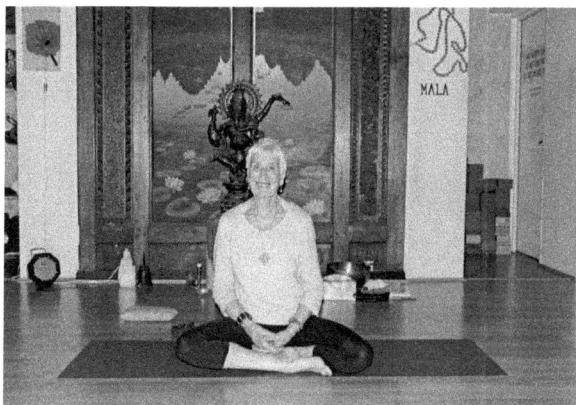

Sheila at Twisting Fish Yoga Studio

Sheila's
Life journey
Is teaching yoga.
46 years of practice,
To a new journey
From England
To Perth.

Sheila teaches yoga at Twisting Fish Studio in Claremont, Perth. The studio is in the middle of the local shopping precinct, which by a twist of fate happened to be around the corner from where I was staying while visiting Perth. My curiosity was immediately piqued as the timetable listed Sheila's classes as specifically for seniors over 65. Walking through the front door of Twisting Fish was like entering another realm – an oasis of calm which seemed a million miles away from the frenetic retail activity and noise of the surrounding shops.

The Tuesday morning class was exactly what I needed that day, slow-paced and gentle. The students had numerous conditions to cater for, including one person with a fractured foot, and another recovering from hip replacement surgery. But nothing was a bother for Sheila – she suitably modified the poses for individual students with ease. The two-hour class flew by and during relaxation at the end, Sheila shared a special contemplative reading, saying, 'Wilfred Clark, the founder of the British Wheel of Yoga, wrote this for me when I first started teaching 46 years ago. I was lucky to have him as my teacher because he was pure yoga itself.'

Sheila was a perfect candidate for my book project, and she agreed to an interview after her next scheduled class, on the upcoming Thursday morning. The class felt special, as if it was customised just for me – and in a way it was. Sheila lovingly tailors her classes to meet the experiences and needs of her students. This class included the 'Rishikesh sequence' which I had never practised before. Sheila later told me, 'I was uncertain whether you were familiar with the Rishikesh, so I took a chance, as I felt it would be a lovely, restorative practice that you could introduce to your own yoga students.' And what a thoughtful gift it was. The Rishikesh[38] *consists of a series of nine essential asanas, performed in a specific order, to work through the whole body and restore balance, as follows:*

Shoulder stand; plough; fish:

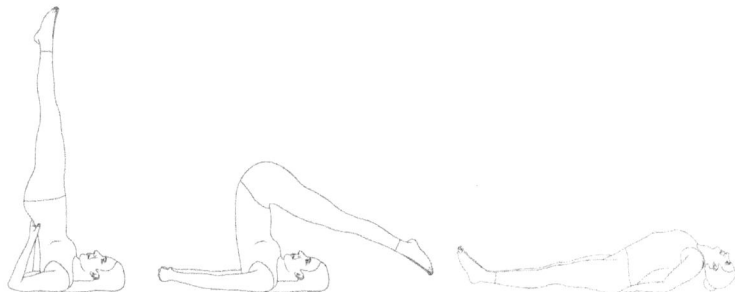

Forward bend; cobra; locust:

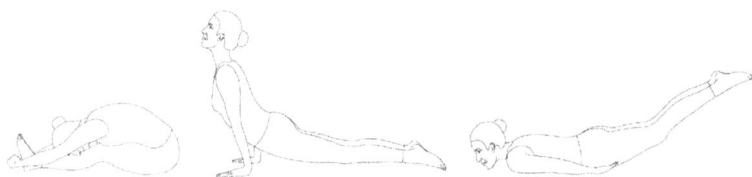

Bow; spinal twist; headstand:

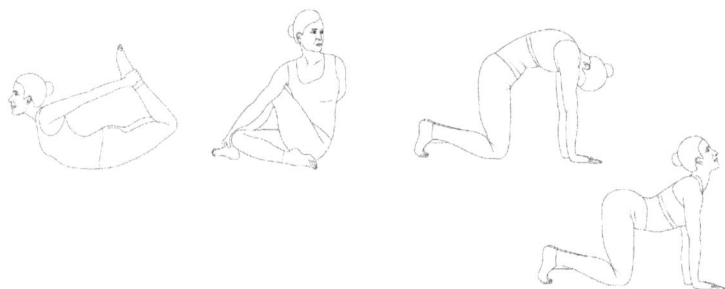

Sheila's instructions also provided a modified version of the Rishikesh to cater for the medical conditions of the students in class – sans headstand (as shown, which was replaced with cat-cow pose to gently massage the spine and belly).

Sheila told me that never in her wildest dreams did she imagine that at the age of 86 she would end up teaching yoga in Australia, after a lifetime spent in England. She moved to Perth five years ago. Her story of what went before, and how it came to pass, follows.

SHEILA'S STORY

Back to the very beginning

My husband worked for the Royal Air Force, and in the late 1960s we were posted to London. A researcher from the local television station happened to have his son at the same school as our two boys. I was chatting with him at the school sports day when, out of the blue, he asked me if I was interested in yoga.

'Well, I don't know much about it,' I replied. 'My husband was educated in India and my father was in the army there. I know yoga comes from India but that's about the extent of my knowledge.'

'The reason I'm interested,' he said, 'is because we're starting a television program about yoga.' Then he added, 'Would you like to come along to a preview and give us your opinion about the show?'

I went along to the television studio in London and met the

director and cast. The program was called *Yoga for Health* and was hosted by an American yoga teacher called Richard Hittleman. Most television programs in those days were broadcast in black and white, but Yoga for Health was transmitted in colour. The visual impact of Richard's two assistants, Cheryl Fischer and Lynn Marshall, dressed in brightly coloured leotards and matching tights was instantaneous! They were both ballet dancers and demonstrated a series of straightforward, easy to follow poses.

As I watched the preview, I thought, *Yes, yoga is what I've been looking for.* I was never interested in performing complex physical movements or participating in competitive sport, but I thought, *I could do yoga.* I had been asked for my opinion though, and the two women demonstrating the poses looked quite young, probably in their early twenties. So, I suggested to Richard that it might be good to have someone a little bit older demonstrating the poses for his show. As soon as I mentioned my idea, I thought, *he thinks I'm referring to myself,* even though that was not my intent as I hadn't yet tried yoga. Anyway, Richard didn't take up my idea. When the program was officially launched in 1970, it was one of the first series broadcast about yoga on British television[39] and ran for five years, taking yoga into people's lounge rooms across the UK.

After watching the preview, I attended a yoga class, but didn't enjoy it. It was the era of hippy *Flower Power.*[40] The whole yoga room reeked of incense, and we walked around and around in circles chanting. I thought, *No way, I don't want to go down this road.* So that was the extent of my venture into yoga, at least for a while. Then the Royal Air Force transferred us to Plymouth in south-west England. I saw an advertisement in an adult education brochure about yoga, and once again went along to a class. This time I enjoyed it because it was practical and down-to-earth. After I attended classes for about a year, my teacher, said, 'Sheila you should teach yoga.'

'Yes, I've considered it,' I replied.

'Splendid, I have two small children,' she added, 'so I don't want to keep teaching in the evening. Will you take over the class for me?'

That's how I started teaching yoga. There were already three other teachers in Plymouth but my classes were always full!

The British Wheel of Yoga

Wilfred Clark was one of the key people who facilitated my deeper involvement with yoga, and for that I'm eternally grateful. Wilfred is renowned for setting up the British Wheel of Yoga in 1965.[41] In the early 1970s, he wanted to expand the Wheel from its initial membership base in Birmingham, to form a network of people across Britain. Unbeknown to me, Wilfred lived in the same town as my godmother (Solihull in the West Midlands), and I had mentioned him in our conversations about yoga. Anyway, my godmother phoned me one day and asked, 'What was the name of that yoga gentleman you wanted to meet?'

'Wilfred Clark,' I replied.

'He lives here, in Solihull,' she said. 'I've seen an advert in the local paper inviting people who are interested in yoga to write to him.'

This was great news. I sent Wilfred a letter and soon afterwards travelled to Solihull to meet him. My serious yoga journey started from that point on.

Once Wilfred had compiled a list of people who were interested in his mission, he organised a group meeting in London. I spent a lot of time going back and forth from Plymouth to London for a series of discussions about how to put yoga on a more official footing. One of the problems was that many British yoga teachers lacked appropriate knowledge and teaching skills. The majority of people, including me, were just thrown into yoga teaching if they could do a few poses; it was basically a case of sink or swim, and 'on the job' learning. To address this deficit, the British Wheel of Yoga (BWY) developed a formal teacher training course. I was a student on their very first course, which was launched in London in 1971.

The standard of the BWY training was first-rate (and still is, entailing a total of 500 hours of work) and back then covered ten subjects, to be completed over a two-year period. Undertaking the course was a substantial commitment as I had two young sons to care for. These days some components of this course are taught online, but back then I had to go up to London every three weeks for my training. While I was away my husband would look after our boys. I was fortunate because he supported me the whole way through the course. It was an exciting time for me, to be there at the beginning when yoga was growing in popularity in the UK – and I relished learning and teaching.

As acceptance of yoga increased in the west, swamis from India started to visit the UK on teaching tours, and one of these,

Swami Shivapremananda (whom I first met in 1971), became the foremost teacher of the BWY for many years. He was a dedicated and exacting teacher, who corrected numerous details of my yoga practice. 'You could do that pose much better,' he would say, or: 'You are not as good as you believe you are – you need to improve.'

At first, I was annoyed and didn't appreciate his critiques of my teaching. I assumed because my classes were popular that I was pretty good at yoga. But once I started to accept his suggestions, I learnt a lot and my teaching certainly improved. One day Swami Shivapremananda said to me, 'You have a lot of work to do, young lady' and I thought, *Oh, here we go again, he's pulling me up about the way I'm practising yoga.* But he continued, 'You're going to start teaching training schemes in the south-west of England.'

I wondered what on earth he was talking about, but strangely enough, some years later that is exactly what I ended up doing.

Yoga in south-west England

In the mid-1970s, the chief inspector for adult education came to meet with me, in my capacity as the BWY representative for south-west England. The local educational authorities were being inundated with requests to run yoga classes, but there was a shortage of qualified teachers – demand was outstripping supply. The chief inspector asked me to train some of the adult education tutors to teach yoga. I agreed to his request, but before the training program could commence, the local education manager needed to endorse its content. 'I will approve a training program in Plymouth and Devon,' he said, 'but I don't want you to include *any* meditation as part of the course.'

I found out that the manager was anti-meditation because of an odd experience he'd personally encountered: he'd been in a class with his wife, and the meditation teacher had directed them to crawl around the room on their hands and knees, and gaze into other students' eyes – on the pretext of revealing their 'true selves'. The manager said to me, 'Yoga teachers are not professionally qualified to deal with any deep-seated issues that might arise for people during meditation practice. Sheila, I hope I haven't offended you?'

'Not at all,' I replied, 'I understand – you're right to be cautious.'

Meditation is often claimed as a panacea for depression. Yet someone with depression is always looking inwards, and meditation accentuates this tendency rather than tempering it. Back in the 1970s, very few people teaching meditation had medical qualifications or counselling skills. Aside from this, yoga teachers only had limited knowledge about the circumstances of their students' lives outside their classes.

My role as the BWY representative also involved working with other local representatives who were based across the UK. We pooled our resources to organise speakers and workshops about yoga. For instance, the regional representative from Wales might phone and say, 'Sheila, a swami from India is visiting Wales at the end of next month, and I know you'd love to have him in the south-west as well.' We would then coordinate the visit, so I'd organise a Saturday seminar in Plymouth, and afterwards we could travel down to Cornwall (the next county) and hold a workshop there the following day. I felt lucky to have those experiences: organising yoga training sessions, meeting interesting people, learning about yoga from swamis and having them stay with my family. I often wondered what our next-door neighbours thought when they saw these men coming and going in their orange robes. Probably something like, *My goodness – Sheila and Jim and their yoga – what are they up to now?*

Jim was in his element because, as I mentioned earlier, he'd spent his childhood in India, and was knowledgeable and enthusiastic about yoga. Although Jim worked full-time, he attended all my evening classes. He'd also regularly visit the local library to do research on yoga and then, based on what he found, make wonderful suggestions for topics or themes to include in my classes. 'You could talk about the *chakras* in the Wednesday night class,' he might suggest, 'but the Friday students probably aren't quite ready for that topic yet.'

On numerous occasions, the swamis who stayed with us advised Jim not to allow me to become overly devoted to any one swami.

'Why?' Jim asked.

'Because Sheila doesn't need a guru – Sheila has yoga within her. Let her gather the information she requires from many people.'

Can you believe that I was sitting there in the same room while the swamis had these sorts of conversations with my husband? In any case, I followed their advice and have never regretted it; I never had a guru, but blended and absorbed the knowledge from different swamis and teachers which resonated within me – and this worked well.

Vegetarianism and my children

Despite growing up surrounded by people dedicated to yoga, my boys didn't get involved with it. They were probably tired of constantly seeing me in a leotard with a yoga mat tucked under my arm. For a while they also suffered the imposition of their parents' commitment to a yogic lifestyle. Out went the meat, white sugar and bread, and in came the brown bread and lentils. One day, an acquaintance said to me, 'Sheila, you're always saying how you prefer to hear the truth about situations. Is that correct?'

'Yes,' I replied.

'Well, I saw both your sons eating hamburgers!'

Jim and I talked it through, and I thought, *We don't have the right to impose this diet on our sons.* Our eldest son, Robert, was about to board at university and in those days, universities didn't have any 'know-how' about vegetarianism – I was worried that he'd be served beans and salad for every meal. So, I told Robert that he needed to include animal protein as part of his diet; and if he wanted to become vegetarian later on, that would be his own choice. I gradually brought animal protein back into our diets, although even today I don't eat much meat.

Another time, our other son, James, returned home all excited from a birthday party. 'Oh, it was awesome, Mum,' he said, 'we had white bread and jam sandwiches!' And I thought, *What have I done to my kids?* Thankfully, they are now normal, well-balanced adults.

A new start – moving to Australia

My life in Plymouth was active and fulfilling. I was happy teaching yoga, and giving talks to various groups about caring for people with Alzheimers; in fact, my husband had developed Alzheimers and I was his carer for ten years. People liked to hear about my personal experiences as a carer: the challenges and rewards, and the importance of asking for help if the responsibility was wearing you down. Despite the difficulties there were many humorous situations that I recall. We were going out one day and Jim had two odd socks on. I said, 'Darling you can't go out wearing odd socks.' He looked down at his feet and said, 'Yes,' then proceeded upstairs to change. But when he came back down, he'd put on the other odd socks from both original pairs!

Then Jim died. One of my yoga students gave a eulogy at Jim's funeral. He had discussed the content beforehand with our sons, Robert and James. At the service, he said, 'Although we [referring to Robert and James] loved our mother and father, we were tired of watching Jim and Sheila down on the floor. They were always in different positions – oh, I am talking about *yoga*!' It was a perfect tribute to Jim because all the people attending the funeral knew our life together revolved around yoga.

After Jim died, I decided to move to Perth (Australia) to live closer to one of my sons (my other son lives in America). It was heart-wrenching saying goodbye to my students. I had taught one of the women for 46 years! I prepared some farewell notes to read out at the end of the last class, but it was so overwhelming I just burst into tears instead.

Fortunately, I started teaching again two weeks after arriving in Perth. How that came about was through my daughter-in-law. She was meeting a friend for coffee and mentioned that I was moving to Australia and taught yoga. 'Well, my partner would be interested in meeting Sheila,' her friend said. It turned out that her partner, Matthew, owned Twisting Fish Yoga Studio in Perth. Matthew came to meet with me soon after I arrived in Australia, and after our initial chat, he asked, 'Would you do me the honour of coming to teach at my studio?'

That was five years ago, and I've been teaching at Twisting Fish ever since.

The nuts and bolts of teaching yoga

Even after 46 years of teaching I still prepare lesson plans because it's important for me to organise classes based on the students' conditions and needs. For instance, the shoulder stand is contraindicated for students with very high blood pressure, as it could aggravate their condition. Another student might be pregnant, which is a specialised area of teaching with numerous precautions. Last week after class, one of my students with osteoporosis said, 'Sheila, I've only been coming to your classes for three weeks, but this is the safest I've ever felt in a yoga class.' And this is what yoga is all about. As students leave my class, I want them to think, *I feel great – this class catered for me.*

Although a deeper understanding of how to work with different students' ailments comes from experience, I believe that yoga teachers need a strong grounding in anatomy and physiology. I was taught this topic as part of the BWY training by Dr Frank Chandra. Aside from being a yoga teacher, he had high level qualifications in medicine and physiology. When I assessed students for their teacher qualifications, some of them made very odd statements about the way they thought the body functions. A classic example was: 'You can tap the various parts of your lungs to breathe.' At the time I thought, *Is this student serious?* Yoga teachers instruct all sorts of people, including doctors and nurses, who will assume on hearing this sort of patter that yoga teachers are ignorant about anatomy and physiology.

In all my years of teaching I've only encountered one student who was disruptive in class. This lady lived nearby but she was always late – arriving just as the other students were starting to relax – and announcing (in a loud voice), 'There's someone in *my* space; *I* always go there.' Or in the middle of class she would make rude remarks about the music, for example, 'I prefer the music you played last week; it's much nicer than today's.' Eventually I had to say to her (as pleasantly as possible), 'You and I need to have a little talk because you're not very subtle. Perhaps you should find another teacher who suits you better.' At about the same time she grew tired of yoga and decided to attend 'keep fit' classes instead. But she was the only problematic student I came across, and her behaviour had to be addressed because it disturbed everyone else.

I am curious about what motivates people to practise yoga,

because I believe students come to class for a reason – although, at first, they may not be consciously aware of what they're seeking. If you asked me, when I started yoga, what I was hoping to find, I would have replied, 'Nothing.' So, I designed a questionnaire on this topic, which I ask new students to fill out. The results have been interesting. No-one ever writes, *I've come to do Salute to the Sun.* The responses are all about *relaxation* or *finding myself.* And finding meaning and direction in life is the true purpose of yoga. In my view, the Eight Limbs of Yoga[42] provides a guide, outlining the steps and boundaries along the way for living a meaningful life. It's difficult to know how much of these basic tenets of yoga to include in classes. In discussing this aspect with other teachers, they rightly acknowledge that there is insufficient time to cover all this material in the one-hour classes they teach. And of course, not all students are interested in exploring this side of yoga. Some just want to do a series of poses and relaxation, then go home. But other students are inquisitive about the background history and philosophy of yoga, so I try to mention an element of this at least once a week in class. In Plymouth, I led a discussion class for students who were interested in exploring these topics.

My aim has always been to make yoga accessible for ordinary people like me: mums, dads, professionals and seniors – people who are not gymnasts or dancers or physically flexible – so they can enjoy the thrill of improved body movement and then leave class feeling good. Sometimes I think: *There are so many yoga teachers out there now. I wonder if people look at me still teaching at my age and say, 'Oh my, she's 80-plus', rather than, 'Oh, look at all the experience she has to offer teaching yoga.'*

I can honestly say I've never, ever been bored teaching yoga. Not once have I woken up in the morning and thought, *Oh no, it's Tuesday class today.* Yoga has been my life journey and I've never regretted a single moment of it.

REFLECTIONS

After the interview with Sheila, I rushed to Perth Airport to catch my flight home. My schedule was a little tight given the unexpected interview with Sheila, but it was a delightful add-on to my trip. However, I made it onto my flight with time to spare. Buckled up and ready for take-off, I pondered Sheila's wisdom from nearly half a century of teaching yoga.

When Sheila first tried yoga, it was an incense-scented, hippie-habit linked to the counter-culture movements of the 1960s, and heavily associated with hippies, drugs and alternative lifestyles. While working in the adult education system, Sheila was advised to call herself a 'keep fit' teacher rather than a 'yoga teacher' – an imperative in situations where her students were married to policemen!

Today yoga is mainstream: there is a yoga studio on every corner, a teacher in every gym, and you can buy a yoga mat at Woolworths or Kmart. Sheila was there right at the start, as yoga entered the west. Demand for yoga teachers outpaced supply, and she was tasked with training increasing numbers of teachers to fill that demand. In contrast, these days yoga teaching is such a popular job that the supply of teachers outpaces demand, and it's getting harder and harder to make a living from teaching yoga.

During class, I assumed that Sheila's extensive knowledge and experience explained her seamless catering to the students' complex ailments and conditions. While partly true, there was so much more to it than this. As Sheila explained, each week she devises a thorough lesson plan: excluding any asanas which might aggravate specific conditions, working out modifications, and searching for something special to include in class – just as she did for me with the Rishikesh sequence. It's no wonder that her students feel safe in her hands, and that her classes are devised especially for them.

Sheila also drew attention to the pervasive idea in the west that yoga is essentially asanas, or bending the body into poses. For her, yoga offers so much more. She embodies yoga philosophy, adding depth and dimension to her teaching, although in the modern, fast-paced world of yoga it is difficult to incorporate this information in classes. And she recognises that not everyone wants a five-minute dharma talk at the start of class, or an explanation of how a sutra links to asana.

On balance, I believe that a great yoga teacher like Sheila will light the lamp of self-inquiry and inspire students to lead richer, healthier and fuller lives. As the swamis had said in England, 'Sheila has yoga within her' – such a teacher may choose to use philosophy for this purpose, or perhaps never utter a Sanskrit word.

#8
LIZ COON

A YEARNING TO EXERCISE

Every single day I am grateful ~ because yoga
gave me back my health

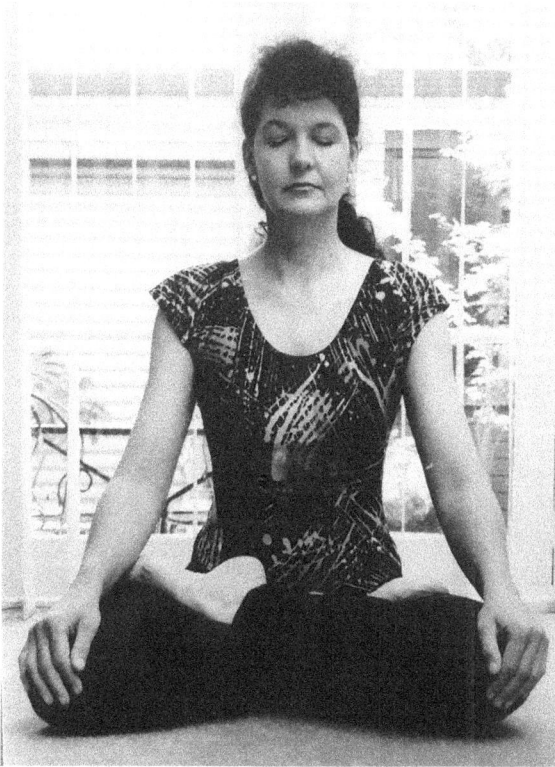

Liz Coon

Kathy Arthurson

Liz Coon
Loves Yoga.
40 years teaching,
Therapeutic health-giving.
Lessening our pain,
Gives so much
Kind soul.

As I climbed the stairs to Liz Coon's Harmony School of Yoga, the melodic sounds of children's laughter drifted from below. The yoga studio was on the first floor, directly above the Syndal Swimming Centre, at Mt Waverley, in suburban Melbourne. At the front desk, Liz's husband, Norm, greeted me warmly. He assists Liz with administrative tasks, including booking in students, taking payments, setting up the yoga room, and organising morning tea after Friday morning classes. This enables Liz to concentrate on teaching. I immediately thought, 'It's a marriage made in yoga.' Liz told me later it wasn't always this way. When she started teaching yoga in the 1980s, many of her friends considered yoga a bizarre practice. With a smile playing across her face she added, 'Even Norm, who is now a yoga enthusiast, for many years called it my hobby.' On the contrary, as Liz reveals in this chapter, for her, yoga has always been a serious vocation.

I attended the Friday morning therapeutic and restorative yoga class. The focus was on nurturing and healing the body, and incorporated a delightful relaxation with the theme of 'letting go of the past'. The two hours flowed by like a joyful dream. After class there was morning tea with the students, who were curious as to why Liz was being interviewed and asked me lots of questions.

Liz and I held the interview afterwards, sitting on the podium in her yoga studio. Although we hadn't met before, we share a mutual link to the Gita School of Yoga. Gita was the first full-time yoga school established in Australia – opening its doors, in Melbourne, in 1954. I completed my yoga teacher training at Gita, and Liz was mentored by its founder, Margrit Segesman. They had both become devotees of yoga and relaxation after using the practices to improve their health.[43]

Here's more about Liz's story of her journey with yoga, including her remarkable connection to Margrit Segesman.

LIZ'S STORY

Longing to move my body

My story about finding yoga starts from experiencing a serious childhood illness. At the age of five I contracted rheumatic fever – it's an inflammatory disease which can cause heart damage. My parents feared the worst, as around the same time a neighbour's son, who was in my class at school, died from rheumatic fever.

As a child I was highly strung and prone to tantrums. It was probably normal behaviour for a five-year-old, but when I contracted rheumatic fever my outbursts needed quelling to prevent further strain on my heart. It might sound odd but the family doctor put me into a semi-comatose state for six months while my mother cared for me at home. After that time, I could sit up and engage in quiet activities like reading, but I still had to stay in bed for another 12 months. This was a commonly prescribed treatment to prevent over-activity and avoid the possibly fatal result of acute heart disease. Not surprisingly, throughout my formative years, I yearned to exercise, but was warned not to because of the damage rheumatic fever had done to my heart.

When I was five, the doctor suggested that I attend a convent school rather than a public school, as the effects of rheumatic fever can last for many years and I needed constant observation during my convalescence. I recall the nuns at the school looked after me very well. While I was at convent school, one of the nuns delivered more distressing news to me about my illness. 'You can never have children,' she said, 'because pregnancy and childbirth would put too much strain on your weakened heart, and you will probably not live past the age of 30 anyway.' Years later this was refuted when I went through childbirth without thinking twice about it. And here I am alive and well in my sixties! Nevertheless, for many years my family bore the scars of my childhood illness. Whenever I was involved in some sort of activity, they would say things like, 'Liz, should you be doing this?'

And I would simply reply, 'Yes, it's no problem at all.'

However, I couldn't exercise in ways that other people took for granted; my heart just couldn't cope and I didn't have enough lung power. For instance, I couldn't walk quickly, or uphill, or do workouts in a gym.

But then yoga came into my life.

When I was about 22 and living in Victoria, I noticed an advertisement for yoga classes in the local paper. I had no idea what yoga was – no inkling whatsoever that it involved exercise – yet the idea intrigued me. So, I went along to a class and was instantly captivated. There was no over-exertion of the body, no jumping up and down or running around. All the poses were done sitting or lying on the floor, and due to these attributes, I could manage it very well. The class was traditional *Hatha Yoga*, held at the then Eastern School of Yoga (at Mt Waverley). The teacher, Mrs Brownrigg, was a firm but wonderful teacher and I went along to her class every day.

As I progressed with yoga and *pranayama* (breathing exercises), my health steadily improved. I believe yoga strengthened my lungs and heart, and built up my physical stamina. I still catch an occasional virus or head cold, but I've never been seriously sick since contracting rheumatic fever as a child. I tell people, 'I'm as fit as a fiddle!' from many years of practising yoga.

Finding Gita

I attended Mrs Brownrigg's classes for about two years. By then I yearned to know more about yoga and wanted to deepen my practice. And that's why in 1977, in my mid-twenties, I decided to train as a yoga teacher. Mrs Brownrigg wouldn't take me on as a trainee because she felt I just hadn't been going to classes long enough. So I found another teacher to train me, Marjorie Marsh from the International Yoga Teachers Association (IYTA). The extent of my training consisted of attending yoga classes and meeting with my teacher once a month. I found that attending classes as a student is a very different experience to teaching yoga; when I began teaching classes the following year, in my lounge room, I was so studious and afraid of doing something wrong that I read the whole class word for word, straight from a book. Today this kind of teaching style would be unacceptable. However, this was only the very beginning of my teacher training, as I then discovered the Gita School of Yoga and I felt like I'd found my way home.

The first time I heard about the Gita School of Yoga (known simply as 'Gita') was when I was working for a group of doctors in Mount Waverley. The patients there kept mentioning this tough woman who taught at Gita – who I later learned was the yoga school's founder, Margrit Segesman. They would say things like, 'Oh, she's scary, you don't want to go there.' For some reason their comments intrigued me, and I absolutely *had* to go to Gita. The classes were always scheduled when I was working evenings at the clinic, so I approached one of the doctors about my dilemma. 'I really want to attend a Gita yoga class,' I said, 'so, I want Monday nights off.'

Much to my surprise, he replied, 'Of course Liz, go ahead.'

The week I finally went to a class, I found out that Margrit Segesman had retired from teaching at Gita, and I was so disappointed. It was 1983, and Di Lucas and Lucille Wood were taking over the management of Gita. A special ceremony called the *Transference of Light* was held to mark the occasion, and it was there that I initially caught a glimpse of Margrit. My first thought was, *I must meet this lady*. However, several years would pass before we met.

In the meantime, I settled in at Gita, and attended classes five days a week. Margrit's 'Gita Yoga' system was better than any other method I had experienced – and I loved it! Gita works through the entire endocrine system, using a series of ten traditional *asanas*, including variations, and is perfect for every body type. I continued to attend Gita for about five years and also started esoteric studies, which is essentially yoga philosophy, and that became my main interest. Unfortunately, the timetable for the esoteric class kept changing during this period, and consequently I ended up repeating the beginner's class three times in a row! Although I learnt a huge amount, it did feel as if I was repeating the basics over and over again.

One day, I heard on the grapevine that Margrit was teaching students at her home. For some unknown reason, I still felt compelled to meet her, so I decided to phone her to talk about my situation. Margrit wasn't rude, but her manner was firm, when she asked, 'Why can't you go to Gita for your studies?'

My immediate thought was, *she's not going to take me on as a student,* but I dug my heels in and replied. 'Well look, the timetable for esoteric classes keeps changing, and it doesn't fit in with my work commitments anymore. And I also teach yoga.'

'Okay,' she said, 'I'll meet with you.'

On the day of our scheduled meeting I knocked on Margrit's front door but another woman answered. 'Who are you?' she asked.

'I'm Liz; I have an appointment with Miss Segesman.'

'Right, stay there and I'll see.' And the door banged shut, right in my face!

I thought, *Oh dear, what have I let myself in for?*

A few minutes went by while I stood outside, and then the door re-opened. This time the woman's manner was totally different and she invited me in. Margrit was ill, and sitting on a chair in her dressing gown. She apologised profusely because she'd forgotten about our meeting – which explained why the woman who answered the door wasn't expecting me. We sat and chatted for a while and something clicked between us. As a result, I started attending two study groups with her. Our time together was the most extraordinary gift for me, and Margrit became my dearest friend. In fact, I eventually became one of her carers, right through to the moment she passed away. She would sometimes ask, 'Why do you stay with me?' It was hard to understand because I appeared out of nowhere into her life. But deep down we both knew it was a 'karmic' connection – we'd been together before, in past lives.

When I initially sought Margrit's advice about studying teacher training at Gita, I'd already done three other yoga training programs. She said to me, 'You don't need to do any more training – just get on with teaching. In fact, Liz,' and she *never* called me Liz, but on this occasion she did, 'you should start your own teacher training program.'

I told her I couldn't possibly do that, but she pushed me to get it started. Due to Margrit's advice and guidance, I started my own yoga teacher training program in 1990, and I'm so grateful to her.

The broad scope of my teacher training courses

Since 1990, I've trained around 52 yoga teachers, most of whom have gone on to teach. It's a two-year course with a prerequisite of two years yoga practice. Some of the trainees were very introverted when they started my course and it was wonderful watching them develop and grow in self-confidence.

Where applicable, I always ask for an interview with the

trainee's partner, because it's important for them to understand the high level of commitment required to successfully complete the course. Specifically, towards the end of the two-year mark, the trainees need to spend a lot more time at the yoga studio. Problems can arise if their partners aren't aware beforehand that they may see less of them than is usual at this time.

Of course, these days you can become a yoga teacher after completing a six-month or even a six-week course. In my view, this is an 'add water and stir' approach to make an instant yoga teacher, who is permitted, without in-depth training, to teach students with injuries or a myriad of other special needs. It does concern me where this approach to teacher training is heading. When people tell me they're doing a quick course to become a yoga teacher, I very kindly say, 'Look it's your choice, but bear in mind that you must be responsible for *how* you teach, and what may possibly happen to your students as a result.'

When I train people as teachers, they're required to experience and explore a variety of different styles of yoga for one month, which means attending classes and observing how yoga is taught by a range of teachers. In one of my groups, all the younger trainees explored Bikram Yoga.[44] After the first class they weren't planning to continue, but the Bikram studio offered low-cost, unlimited introductory classes – just $19 for two weeks. So, my students decided to take up the offer and said to me, 'We might as well get our $19 worth.' They then became immersed in Bikram Yoga. Once they finished my training, some of these students undertook the Bikram teaching training. Two from that group are now running Bikram studios. I've also had students leave my studio because I don't teach Vinyasa Yoga.[45] I'm not disturbed by this: in my view, it's important for everyone to experience different styles of yoga to discover what suits them best.

Dealing with death and dying as a yoga teacher

During the 1990s, many terminally ill people came to see me: they found me through my newspaper advertisements for meditation, relaxation and yoga. I offered each topic as a stand-alone class. These students were mainly interested in meditation or receiving a healing through the classes. Explaining to them that the practices might not restore their health was truly heart-wrenching for me. Many of these people were suffering from terrible afflictions but, as it turned out, they all became my dear friends – and I was with most of them when they passed, according to their wishes.

The first time one of these friends passed while I was present, it was in the pre-dawn hours. Afterwards I decided to visit Margrit Segesman as her house was on my way home, and I knew she'd be awake early. I made Margrit a cup of coffee and asked, 'Why do you think he wanted me to stay with him at the end?'

'Because in a way you're like a priest – all yoga teachers are,' she said.

I hadn't thought about it in this way before, but Margrit was right: people disclose all sorts of information to their yoga teachers. Therefore, it's important to be ethical when you teach yoga. Every day I check in with myself to ensure I'm treating each person in front of me as an individual and taking them seriously – even if I'm busy or distracted, I never want to become flippant.

Eventually I had to stop seeing so many seriously ill people. It was difficult dealing with so much suffering and dying. I was becoming worn down trying to cope with it all, especially as difficult circumstances were arising in my own personal life. In 1997, one of the yoga teachers at my studio contracted leukaemia, and upon visiting her one day, I found she had lapsed into a coma. The following year, I was with my dear friend, Margrit Segesman, when she passed away. Then my daughter, who was also a yoga teacher, suffered a life-threatening stroke; this was followed by my sister requiring surgery. On and on these traumatic events went, until it reached the point where I pulled back and said, 'Stop. I've had enough. I need to step away.' It's not that I don't see people who are unwell anymore, because I still do. But these days I've learnt how to help people without allowing it to deplete me.

Adjusting my own yoga practices

After my daughter's illness I also had to reorganise my other routines. For many years my meditation practice was at 3 a.m. because all my teachers advised me to meditate at that time. At first it was a challenge, and if I overslept, I decided not to give myself a hard time; I just accepted what happened and said to myself, *Okay, I'll try to do better tomorrow.* When I did manage to get up at 3 a.m. I'd do a one-hour meditation practice, followed by some yoga or esoteric study. After that, I was ready to go to work. In those days I had boundless energy: I never went to bed much before midnight and would get up fighting fit after just three hours sleep. These days, when I meditate, it's usually at 5 a.m., and sometimes after a long, tiring day I fall asleep on the couch. But I still sleep for a limited number of hours – yoga gives me the energy I need.

I also had to adjust my diet, and I'm no longer a purist. For the first 30 years of teaching yoga, I was strictly vegetarian and fasted once a week. I only ate salads or other wholesome food – biscuits, chips or junk food never passed my lips. However, after Tanya suffered the stroke I found myself slipping into McDonald's and buying chips to keep me going. My time was limited as I was caring for Tanya, as well as managing a hectic routine of teaching numerous classes.

Today I've reached an age where I think it's much more important to pay attention to my diet. Several years ago, I started eating meat again, mainly because my daughter felt she needed meat in her diet to gain strength. And clearly this dietary change has helped her. My view about diet is that most things are fine in moderation. For instance, I might put small amounts of meat in a stew to ensure there's enough protein for Tanya. There are also other practicalities to consider, and cooking different types of meals for each member of my family would require 24 hours of daylight! So, one day I simply decided that life is short and there's absolutely no reason to stick to rituals. Many people, and particularly yogis, chastise themselves for not following a vegetarian diet but my reasoning is: if you need to eat meat due to your health or other reasons – what does it matter? I don't give myself a hard time about eating meat but I do feel that it should be prepared ethically.

At a physical level, I've always worked quite hard with my

own yoga practice. When Mr Iyengar, the founder of Iyengar Yoga[46], visited Australia, I attended his classes and found him a precise and wonderful teacher. Although I've been teaching for over 40 years, I still refer to his book, *Light on Yoga*[47] when I need to check specific yoga posture details. In fact, I call this book my 'yoga bible' because his descriptions of the postures are meticulous. Despite this, I personally find the style of Iyengar Yoga too strict. In 2000, I started practising Ashtanga Yoga[48] – and I absolutely love it. Several students who came to my studio told me they'd hurt their backs in Ashtanga classes. I asked them if they knew what had caused this, but they had no idea.

I decided to attend an Ashtanga class to find out what practice might be causing these back injuries, and quickly realised it was during the Salute to the Sun sequence. Specifically, where you jump to the back of the mat, then jump forward. I found that modifying this manoeuvre so that you *step* back and forward, without jumping, works well for people with back issues.

Teaching on and off the mat

The way I teach a yoga class depends on observing how the students are feeling on the day and what they need. It's important to get the right balance for students: the fine line between doing too little and doing too much in a class.

Poses like plank and downward dog are useful and important poses for building strength and bone density, and in downward dog pose it's also easy to notice when a student's body is out of alignment. And while I encourage students to extend themselves within postures, I also advise them to pull back from a stretch if it becomes too much. This discrimination builds their self-awareness towards finding an appropriate balance between taking it too easy and overdoing their practice.

Something I never thought I'd ever do is teach 'off the mat', but that's another way my personal teaching style has changed. Originally, I taught 'on the mat' which means I performed the postures on my mat, simultaneously calling out the movements and instructions for the students to follow. I still teach 'on the mat' in smaller classes, but teaching a big class is not the same: instead of performing *with* the students, a teacher needs to walk around the class to check what the students are doing. My advice for other yoga teachers – especially those who struggle to keep up with the physical demands of teaching – is, 'Don't do all the postures yourself. You can sit on the podium and give your students instructions while you watch. You'll still be a good yoga teacher and at the same time, you won't have to give up teaching if you're struggling physically.'

All up, I teach seven classes a week, not counting private one-on-ones with students. There are occasions when I think, *Oh I don't want to go to the studio today*, but that's just my mind talking. As soon as I get to the studio, I feel truly uplifted; I get so much out of teaching. I also love my students; to be honest, if I didn't teach, I would really miss working with them. I believe that most students come to class for a 'bit of the spiritual side of yoga' along with the other aspects. Although of course, not everyone wants to study esoterics, or yoga philosophy.

It's also a privilege being amongst other yoga teachers and I still learn a lot from these people. As a yoga teacher, my view is that once you stop learning, then it's time to give it up; and keeping up a personal yoga practice is essential if you want to teach effectively. Anyone can teach yoga, but I believe that the ongoing challenge is to teach *well*, with integrity and an open heart.

That's my story of how I became involved with yoga, through experiencing a debilitating childhood illness and finding a way forward. Yoga has been with me for almost my whole life, and every single day I am grateful because it gave me back my health.

REFLECTIONS

After we finished our interview, Liz kindly drove me to the local railway station where we said our goodbyes. As I sat on the train, reflecting on the morning's activities, so many thoughts entered my mind. I found Liz's class so caring and therapeutic – her 40 years of teaching and devotion to yoga shone through. As it was a large class, I also experienced first-hand Liz's 'off the mat' teaching style; she taught the class with grace and ease. All the students benefited, including me, as she walked around checking whether our poses were being performed correctly.

I also found it fascinating that Liz restored her own health through practising yoga. The serious side-effects of her childhood illness are no longer apparent. Now in her sixties, Liz clearly experiences health as a positive state of 'being' with plenty of energy for the full and active life she leads.

The day I started writing up these reflections, I received an email from the owner of a highly respected local yoga studio, informing me that the difficult decision had been made to discontinue their extensive yoga teacher training course. As outlined in the email, they could no longer compete with the vast number of short, cheap training programs on offer, without compromising their own standards – which they were, of course, unwilling to do. As I read the email, I was reminded of Liz's stark illustration highlighting the allure of the 'quick fix' yoga course.

The same week, I had a new student in my yoga class. I asked her about any injuries or other issues I should be aware of when teaching her. She informed me that she had serious knee injuries from completing a short, intensive yoga teacher training course at a resort in Asia. This begs the question: 'Are we starting to see the demise of excellence in yoga teacher training?' In my view, it reinforces the importance of seeking out highly capable teachers, like Liz, and indeed all the teachers in this book, who are committed to a personal yoga practice, ongoing learning and self-development.

⁂

POSTSCRIPT

Written by Liz Coon, in memory of her beloved husband, Norm, who passed away on the 21st April 2017.

As I sit here writing, wonderful memories and impressions flood into my mind of my dear husband, Norm. I remember him looking after the yoga school desk in our studio – and his smiling, sometimes cheeky face as he greeted students. That's what the students loved about Norm, and what they commented on most after he passed away. He was always happy, and they would miss his cheerful greeting as they rushed upstairs to class. They enjoyed confiding in Norm about the things happening in their lives while he listened patiently.

Norm helped me organise the yoga school so that I had time to focus on teaching; assisting with setting up workshops, new classes, teacher training, morning teas and meditations. Each year he would play the role of 'Easter Bunny', bringing hot-cross buns for breakfast after the Good Friday meditation class.

Norm loved golf, enjoyed the horse races and attended six yoga classes (of all levels) every week. He had a dry, wonderful sense of humour and people who knew him well recognised when he was joking or serious, whereas others were sometimes bewildered! He enjoyed meeting all the people who came to yoga classes and often made us laugh. He thoroughly enjoyed life and always made an effort to help – nothing was too much trouble. He helped bring our whole yoga community together and took everything in his stride.

Norm supported, inspired and motivated me whenever I needed it. I love Norm so much, and miss his company, his humour, and his counsel. I miss him just being here. We were a team.

Dearest Norm, thank you for being in my life, and for sharing our love of yoga together.

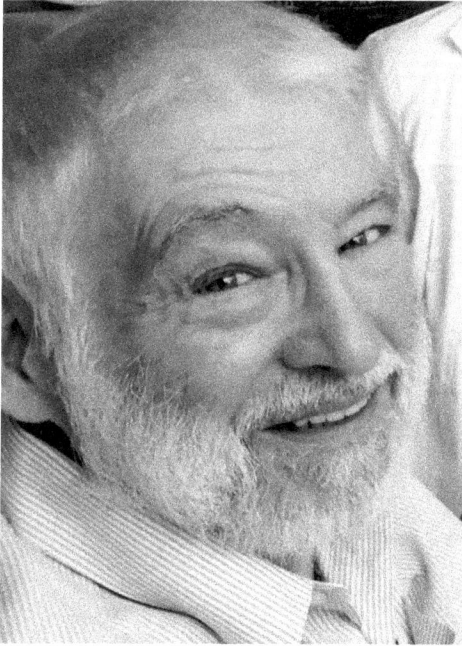

Norm Coon

#9
JUDY MORGAN
(Swami Karmashakti Saraswati)

GIVING THE GIFT OF YOGA

Teaching yoga to people in rural Australia has been
one of the highlights of my life

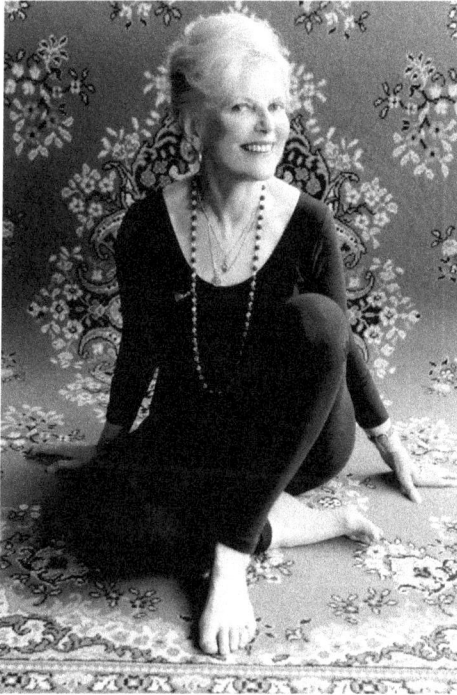

Judy Morgan
(Courtesy Star Newspapers)

Judy
In Penrith,
Yoga is her Gift.
For students on chairs and mats
With her co-teacher.
Brings balance
And calm.

I discovered Judy Morgan's website, Living Beautifully, while browsing the internet in search of yoga teachers to interview for this book. Her photo captivated me – a presentiment of her authentic serenity and warmth.

I participated in Judy's Tuesday morning 'intermediate level' class at the North Penrith Community Centre. The centre is two kilometres from the Penrith central business district, but as the taxi meandered along the lengthy driveway, it was like entering an enchanted forest. Luxuriant trees peppered the grounds surrounding the centre. Judy's class comprised a mix of age groups, including several younger students and others aged 70 plus. We practised some of the stronger, standing warrior poses, but the class was still wonderfully relaxing and meditative.

Judy has taught yoga for 58 years and currently teaches eight classes each week. When I mentioned that this seemed rather a lot, she said, 'Even though yoga gives me lots of energy, at 78 it would be tiring to teach that many classes. So, these days I co-teach with my assistant Sari.' It was a rare treat, experiencing first-hand two accomplished yoga teachers sharing the teaching of a class: taking turns, demonstrating and instructing the poses. As Judy explained, the reason this partnering works marvellously is because they love working together.

Judy and I had our interview after class, in the community centre, over several cups of tea. As we chatted, it was like travelling across time on a fascinating, historical yoga journey. Judy has been involved in yoga since the 1950s, and instrumental in its development in Australia. But, as she expresses in her story, following the path of yoga hasn't always been smooth or easy –

along the way there have been numerous interruptions and lessons
in life – with each challenge taking her from strength to strength.

JUDY'S STORY

Coming to the mat

The very first time I heard the word 'yoga' something awakened inside me. It was in 1956 (when I was 17 and living in Melbourne), and I was chatting to a woman at a social gathering, who started talking about yoga. However, several years passed before I found a yoga class to try and even then, the only class I knew about was at Gita Yoga, in the Melbourne CBD. I approached the centre three times before I was brave enough to go inside, as I was nervous about what might happen. That was my first experience of yoga, but I couldn't continue at Gita because it was such a long way from where I lived. So, I practised on my own at home using the book, *Yoga for Women* (written by prominent yoga teachers, Nancy Phelan and Michael Volin), which taught me so much – in fact, I have read that book from cover-to-cover many times.

When I was 20, I found a yoga teacher called Gloria Christensen, who lived nearby and taught yoga in her lounge room. Previously, she'd been badly injured in a car accident and confined to a wheelchair. But after practising yoga for some time, she was able to start walking again. I was astonished that Gloria had achieved this through yoga. For me Gloria was a lovely teacher, who turned herself 'inside-out' performing a variety of poses. In her classes I discovered I could accomplish the yoga poses, which was exciting as I was never any good at sport. After each class, I'd arrive home and say to my former husband, 'Let me show you the poses I learnt tonight!'

In the early 1960s, my baby son became unwell and needed very expensive medication. As a consequence of the worry and stress around his illness, my own health also deteriorated. Gloria stepped in and gave me the perfect gift: encouraging me to attend more of her yoga classes, free of charge. Her generosity taught me the lesson that I could do the same for other people in need.

Starting to teach

I attended Gloria's classes for about three years. Then one day she asked me to teach a class, to fill in for her, while she went away. I had no teacher training whatsoever, but taught everything I could think of in that one-hour class – until I ran out of poses to do! When I consider this situation now, I think, *Oh my goodness, how on earth did I manage to do that?* Afterwards, Gloria asked me to take over her classes permanently as she was moving to Queensland. I accepted, and in between having another baby, I taught yoga in my lounge room. Soon after, I met a few people at the local golf club who wanted to try 'this funny thing called yoga.' As a result, I started teaching yoga at the golf club, and from the start there were 20 students in the class. My teaching was basic: mostly on the physical level with *asana*, and very little *pranayama* or relaxation – but the students seemed happy with it.

Although the classes were going well, I felt quite lost without a teacher to guide me: there was no one to learn from, share experiences with, or turn to for advice – not a single person. I recall in those early years of teaching, a couple of students remarked, 'Oh, you're far too young to be a teacher.' Of course, if someone said that now I'd be flattered, but back then their comments upset me. So, I decided to phone Michael Volin[49] for advice; we'd never met, but I felt as if I already knew him, as I used his book on yoga for practising and teaching. Michael was incredibly wise and supportive, and I felt much better after our chat.

In the 1960s, a yoga class was a glamourous event, where women wore fishnet stockings, big earrings and leotards. The yoga teachers and students were generally married, stay-at-home mums. For us, yoga was an important social occasion that one dressed up for: I lived in Box Hill and would never, *ever*, go into Melbourne without wearing a hat and gloves.

Yoga in the 1970s

In the 1970s, I moved to Townsville with my family, and became involved with Satyananda Yoga – a style that felt 'right' for me. I also joined the Queensland Yoga Fellowship Association; its president, Ailsa Gartenstein, and I started travelling up to Innisfail and Cairns, then down to Brisbane, with the aim of taking yoga out into the wider community. It was a wonderful experience giving classes, demonstrations and talks on yoga to these different communities. Additionally, I connected with another yoga teacher, June Jackson (as she was known then, now

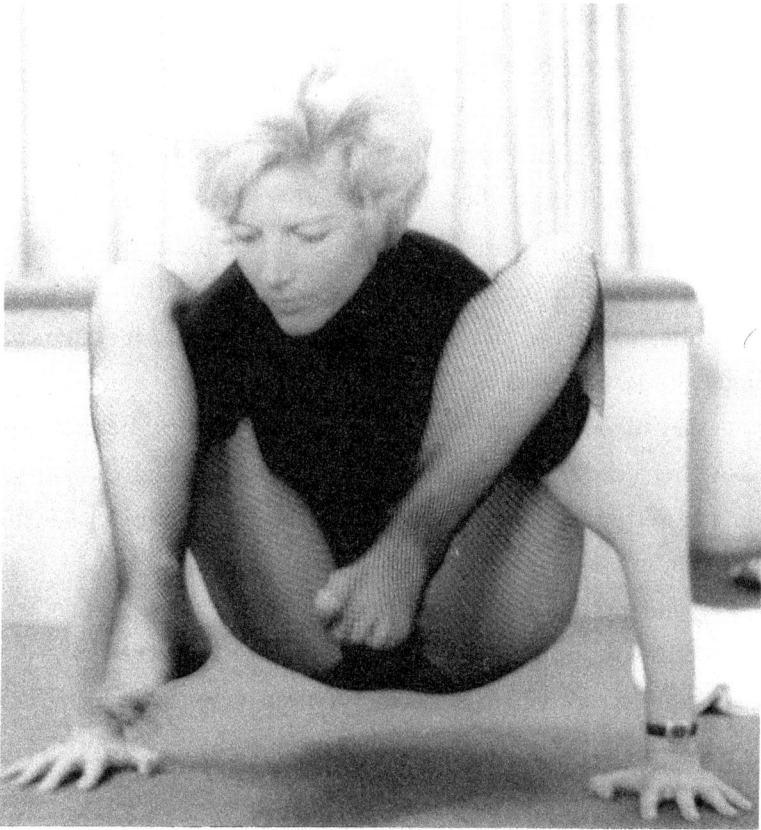

Judy Morgan practising yoga in 1971

Dr June Henry). We organised for a Satyananda swami to visit from India, which was an extraordinary event for the people of Townsville. They had no idea what to expect, but as you can imagine they were incredibly curious. The public lecture and yoga workshop were both very successful, and reported on positively by the local paper and radio station. After this initial success, other swamis started visiting Townsville. It was a magical time in my life: I welcomed various swamis to stay with my family and at the same time, I learnt a huge amount about the practice, background and philosophy of yoga.

Then I was asked to teach yoga in Hughenden, an outback town west of Townsville, and I flew there every second month in a tiny plane called a Fokker Friendship. I taught an afternoon class for the children and an evening class for adults in the local community hall. I recall the tin roof on that hall made it extremely hot! The kind-heartedness of the local people was remarkable, and they always invited me to stay in their homes. Before each visit I recorded a few yoga classes for a local girl – in those days on a cassette tape – and she'd use the tape to organise classes in between my trips.

Several swamis also started to accompany me to Hughenden. In those days, people living in these areas of the outback were extremely receptive to yoga: they craved new experiences and wanted to be part of what was happening in the rest of Australia. This was before information became more widely available on the internet. The whole way we communicate has changed hugely since those days. Personally, I don't feel that having information online is as special or as effective as communicating face-to-face.

By this stage, I had a lot of informal yoga training under my belt. Then in 1973, for the first time I found a formal qualification to undertake – the International Yoga Teachers Association (IYTA) teacher training course. The founder of IYTA, Roma Blair, signed my teaching certificate, which made it extra special! I also taught meditation at the James Cook University in Townsville, which added to my credibility as a yoga teacher.

The 1970s was a 'hippy era' and an opportune time to be involved in yoga, as eastern philosophy and spiritual concepts were reaching wider audiences. In the mid-1970s, a group of school teachers, who were on exchange from the Seattle Education Department (in North America) started attending my classes. When they returned to Seattle, they couldn't find a local Satyananda teacher, so they simply paid my fare and organised for me to teach yoga in Seattle for six weeks.

Always a yogi in your heart

I lived in Townsville for nine years, then my marriage fell apart and I moved to Sydney with my children. Finding a job in Sydney was difficult; I remember talking to one of the Satyananda swamis about it, 'I feel afraid of losing yoga,' I said, 'because I need to start working in a shop, selling cosmetics to earn money.'

'Just do it,' he said to me. 'You'll always be a yogi in your heart – you'll always find ways to keep yoga in your life.'

I believe from that point on, with every step I took, yoga was all around me. I applied for a job with a cosmetic company, and the woman I spoke to on the phone was delighted to hear that I'd been teaching yoga.

'Well, I've just started going to yoga classes!' she said, 'come in for an interview.'

My interview was successful and I was given a job with that company, selling cosmetics. Then the training director also asked me to teach yoga classes in her home. I ended up working as a training director for two companies, as well as teaching yoga.

Sometimes I felt anxious about fulfilling my responsibilities, but I used yoga to 'come back to my centre', to calm my emotions and slow my mind – I would focus on my breath and just 'be me'. It was a very busy period in my life: I also gave public lectures, sometimes to audiences of around 200 people. I found it easy to relate the lecture topics with different aspects of yoga. For example, one of the companies sold skin creams and other products which were 'soothing', so I talked about yogic relaxation.

I did all this for about eight years, and during this time I remarried. My new husband and I were living in Darling Point, which is close to the Sydney CBD, but we wanted to buy our own home and found one that suited us in Penrith. That was 34 years ago, and at the time, we didn't think our move would be permanent because Penrith seemed so far away from Sydney. But we made many wonderful friendships, and I opened a beauty salon in Penrith, which became a successful business (it also mixed very well with teaching yoga). I stopped running the beauty therapy business five years ago as I was getting tired, but I'm still teaching yoga.

Teaching today

One of the things I love most about teaching is seeing friendships develop between people. For some students who live alone, the social aspect is almost as important as the yoga practice. In our morning classes there is always time before and after class to chat, whereas there's only a 15-minute break in between the two evening classes, which leaves little time for socialising. However, most people attending night classes have been at work all day; they're generally tired and want to relax, then slip away after class to attend to other things.

For a long time, my personal yoga practice was very much physically-based with strong postures, but I gradually learnt that yoga didn't need to be so strenuous to benefit my body. Consequently, as I've aged and grown in awareness, my needs have also changed. Increasingly I've turned more to meditative practices and *pranayama*. As a result, I also teach differently. For example, I regularly teach a seniors' group who have their yoga classes seated on chairs. It took me a *year* to get them seated on chairs because they thought 'chair yoga' was only for old people! Now they're practising lots of *pranayama*, as well as the *Pawanmuktasana Series One*.[50] There is a wide range of important practices in yoga, but if I had to choose, I would say Pawanmuktasana is number one, because the simple joint movements, as well as the stretching and warm up exercises, keep the body moving and supple. The students in this class have told me that they find Pawanmuktasana empowering. Interestingly, I never advertised this seniors' class: it was suggested by a friend, who was also the first student in the class and travelled from Sydney to Penrith to attend it. Well, the class just *took off* – more and more students came along, and now the class is always full.

At one stage, I made a good living out of teaching yoga but it's much harder for teachers these days. In the Penrith region alone, up to the top of the Blue Mountains, there are about 60 yoga teachers. Even gyms have yoga teachers, which means that everyone's 'slice of the pie' is much smaller than in previous years.

In the past ten years, I haven't had the best run of health, but in my view how you cope with health issues is important. I'm always positive and recover quickly even after I've had surgery (like my knee replacement). My husband is also a positive person, but he's dealing with cancer and a heart problem. If I didn't have yoga to re-energise me, I think this situation could wear me down. But I can walk away for a while, teach yoga and 'be me' again, then go back and look after him, when he needs my support.

I think as you age, it's very wise, and healthy, to nurture a passion like yoga and to pursue doing what you love – this prevents you from merging into ageing and just growing old. I intend to keep on teaching, but if I become too old to teach and who knows when that might be, I'll continue to mentor yoga teachers. Mentoring is lovely because you see people blossoming, growing, changing and feeling better about themselves.

I have a delightful team around me in my yoga business today. There are five of us, and the others are all much younger than me. Some of these women did their yoga teacher training with me and when they'd finished, they asked if they could stay on to teach. We're like a yoga family – in fact, we call ourselves the *Om Brigade!*

I've been teaching for 58 years, and I still have my own personal practice – along with an enduring passion for yoga. Giving the gift of yoga to people in rural locations, who were keen to practise and learn, has been one of the highlights of my teaching life, and gave me great joy. These experiences remain dear to my heart, and hopefully – through my own practice and teaching of yoga over so many years – others have been as deeply touched. I believe the practice and sharing of yoga helps everyone to live more fulfilling lives, and I'm so grateful to have been part of the spread of yoga throughout the Australian community and beyond, for all these years.

REFLECTIONS

After we finished our interview, Sari (Judy's co-teacher) drove me to Penrith Railway Station. Judy needed to return home to help her husband, who was feeling unwell. As I sat on the train contemplating the morning's visit, a myriad of thoughts came into my mind. I reflected on what Judy had said, about the spirit of co-operation she'd experienced with other yoga teachers in the 1970s: 'We all gathered together, exchanged knowledge and helped each other. It was wonderful and good – pure and true.'

I was also struck by how Judy comes from the Satyananda tradition, which teaches such a beautiful, gentle and wholistic form of yoga: incorporating *asana, pranayama,* relaxation and meditation. In fact, all the teachers featured in this book share that deeper aspect, teaching yoga far beyond a physical focus. The predominantly physical approach to yoga seems to have become more common in contemporary western society. Now we have numerous 'gimmicky' derivatives of yoga: Beer Yoga, Doga (yoga with your dog), even Goat Yoga – all of which have a commercial, competitive and popularised basis, which detracts from yoga as an ancient tradition designed to enhance stability and self-growth in an individual's life.

Talking with Judy also reminded me that it was far too

long since I had practised the Pawanmuktasana series – and by happenstance, a new student turned up at my class who suffers from arthritis. As I worked my way through the Pawanmuktasana series with the students, I realised I'd forgotten just how good these practices feel. The series offers such a simple, low impact method to keep the body healthy and joints moving, in a way which respects tenderness or weakness in the tissues.

I also pondered over what Judy said about her teacher giving her 'the gift of yoga', and how in turn she has shared that gift with others through her own teaching. It reminded me of the following inspirational quote:

> *'The purpose of life is to discover your gift.*
> *The work of life is to develop it.*
> *The meaning of life is to give your gift away.'*[51]

Judy has accomplished all this and more with her gift of yoga.

#10
PRACTISE YOGA

FOR RADIANT AGEING

Dear readers, you might be tempted to think, *wow look at the women in this book – they have spent their lives doing yoga and it has paid off* – but that's not helpful if you haven't practised yoga. Another way of looking at this situation is to ask: what are these women doing right now and what can we learn from them? I leave you thus with my summary of their combined wisdom about vibrant ageing (along with supporting evidence).

1. Take time to relax and practise *pranayama* (yogic breathing).
2. Move your body.
3. Keep learning and doing what you love (and stay happy and contented).
4. Make a choice to age mindfully (and embrace the 'longevity bonus').
5. Focus on 'healthy eating' and make peace with food.
6. Maintain positive social connections.
7. Find the right teacher and style of yoga to suit you.

1. Take time to relax and practise *pranayama* (yoga breathing)

Several months ago, I walked into my favourite café (pondering the final chapter of this book) and spotted this proverb – in big, bold letters – on the memo board:

> *If you don't choose time to rest and rejuvenate – your body will choose it for you*
> *# take care of yourself*

This advice could have been penned by any one of the nine yoga teachers in this collection. They all emphasised the importance of not skimping on yogic breathing and relaxation practices. These are the secret ingredients that differentiate yoga from other forms of exercise – such as, working out in a gym – and lead to practitioners looking younger and more relaxed after attending classes. If you think this sounds fanciful, rest assured that the findings of scientific studies support this notion, pointing to yogic breathing and relaxations as perfect practices for providing balance between the sympathetic and parasympathetic parts of the autonomic nervous system.[52] A balance that is critical for overall health and wellbeing.

The sympathetic nervous system is aroused whenever we are faced with an actual (or perceived) fearful or dangerous situation, pumping the body full of stress hormones (including cortisol) and causing the flight, fight or freeze response. The parasympathetic nervous system performs the opposite: activating the body's calming system (once the threat has passed), quietening the stress hormones and allowing the body precious time to rest and heal. In fast-paced modern life, the sympathetic nervous system is easily over-stimulated. Yogic breathing (diaphragmatic breathing) and relaxation practices alleviate this imbalance, through switching on the calming parasympathetic nervous system. This action decreases cortisol and increases serotonin and melatonin, the marvellous hormones that make us feel happy and relaxed.[53][54]

Hence, just as these teachers advise, yogic breathing and relaxations are simple but wonderful tools (to explore with an experienced yoga teacher) that serve to nurture the body, allowing time to rest, relax, rejuvenate and remedy the stresses of modern life.

2. Move your body

These teachers are also exemplars of the positive impacts of various yoga *asana* (physical poses) on the body and mind. They believe that many unpleasant physical symptoms of ageing are simply due to lack of bodily movement. As you may have already guessed, studies have found that increased physical activity in older adults is indeed associated with lower levels of chronic health problems and illness[55], and higher levels of mental wellbeing and health-related quality of life.[56] The beauty of yoga is that the practices are easily modified to suit recovery from injuries or changes in levels of mobility and fitness at any age. The practice doesn't have to be difficult as there is a smorgasbord of simple movements to choose from, including stretching and warm up exercises to keep the joints moving and body supple; and yoga can even be practised while seated on a chair (a style known as 'chair yoga').

I was astonished at how effortlessly the yoginis in this book can raise themselves from a seated position on the floor. A reduced ability to rise from the floor (for adults aged 51–80) is associated with higher mortality.[57] Sustaining this ability is a critical factor in maintaining age-related independence – otherwise everyday mishaps, like dropping reading glasses onto the floor, can become major challenges. A clear case of the adage 'use it or lose it', and practising yoga can help to maintain this important capability.

3. Keep learning and doing what you love (and stay happy and contented)

The women here have described teaching yoga as giving their lives meaning and purpose as they grow older, providing a source of accomplishment, and a way of contributing to the greater good (that is, through benefiting the health and wellbeing of others beyond themselves). Teaching also requires a range of abilities: maintaining, updating and developing new skills, planning classes, learning new ways of presenting information, communicating with a range of people, along with creativity and problem-solving in catering to the individual needs of students. All these tasks are important exercises for the brain, which are also proven to enhance mental skills as we age.[58] As one of these teachers said, 'when you stop learning it's time to give up being a teacher.'

The philosophical side of yoga has provided these women with guidance and the emotional resilience to 'bounce back' during difficult times, along with a myriad of practices to ease pain and stress, and to deal with the challenges of daily life (such as divorce and death). These women also talked about their yoga teaching (or self-practice) as helping them to develop positive attitudes: becoming more patient, self-aware, kinder, happier and contented with life. These profound benefits of yoga are not reserved for teachers but are strengthened as well in students who regularly attend classes.[59]

When these teachers engage in self-practise they describe a state that psychologists call *being in the flow*. They become unaware of time and are purely in a creative zone. Their minds become totally absorbed in the yoga practice, so thoughts simply drop away, the mind chatter quietens and there is a heightened awareness of the present moment, or in *being here right now*. This 'flow state' has been studied and is indeed found to make us more peaceful, happier and contented human beings.[60]

4. Make a choice to age mindfully (and embrace the 'longevity bonus')

The teachers in this book are relishing the opportunities that come with the 'longevity bonus' (or longer life spans). They don't accept limiting, negative stereotypes that expect older people to act in certain ways. No, on the contrary, these women have invented their own chronicles about growing older – some are still performing headstands (safely) in their 90s – and there is no magic age when they expect to retire from teaching or practising yoga. At the same time, they don't deny the realities of ageing or pretend it's not happening; they *do* accept biological ageing, yet maintain a semblance of control over the process.

The key to this positivity about ageing seems to be the mind-body connection and mindfulness (acceptance and self-awareness) that yoga practices facilitate. Separation between the mind and body as we age (i.e. between the inner-self and thoughts, and the external, physical body) sets up stress, denial, feelings of lack of control, non-acceptance and even anger about age related changes.[61] In these yoginis, their minds and bodies work in harmony – rather than at loggerheads – and their self-talk seems eternally positive. During our interviews, I never heard them say things like, *I'm too old to try something new*. Instead of denying ageing, or just drifting into older age, they are ageing *mindfully* – accepting and respecting what cannot be changed and exploring new ways to stay active and maintain as healthy a body and mind as they possibly can. Where needed, for instance, they have gradually adopted a gentler yoga practice, which is focused more on the inner self (with increased *pranayama* and relaxation) and less on the outer world and harder physical *asana* (poses).

The more people can see all these different ways that one can use their 'longevity bonus' – and when there are a variety of healthful models of ageing – the more attitudes about ageing will change for the better.

5. Focus on 'healthy eating' and make peace with food

Perhaps you are like me and confused about the best foods to eat for optimal health, because dietary choices are associated with life expectancy, lifetime risk for all chronic diseases and gene expression.[62] But what exactly is optimal eating? There is a plethora of diets to choose from: paleo, low fat, low carb, mediterranean, vegetarian, low glycaemic, to mention only a few; some are more rigid than others, but they all exclude specific ingredients. I find it perplexing because there is an absence of conclusive evidence for the superiority of one type of rigid diet over another.[63] [64]

Consequently, I was very interested in these women's views about diet and how it relates to the yogic lifestyle. For most, the solution seemed straightforward, based on a 'healthy eating' approach, characterised largely by a plant-based diet with natural, minimally processed foods (as close to nature as possible). The weight of evidence from different studies about nutrition also suggests a theme of 'healthy eating' works best to optimise health.[65]

Attitude towards food was also mentioned as important, meaning being flexible and not too fixated or rigid about food choices (excluding known allergies and other special requirements). The women pointed out, that our bodily constitutions are unique, and it is often a matter of trial and error with different foods to find what suits each individual best. Most of these yoginis are vegetarians; some have had to accept changes to their diets to reintroduce animal protein for various reasons, including combatting anaemia, or for their children's own changing health needs. Returning to the theme of attitude about food they all advocated *acceptance and not beating yourself up about dietary choices.*[66]

The other word of advice here was to let go of guilt. Personally, I relish this advice! If you indulge in chocolate or a piece of cake, then spend time enjoying the experience rather than tormenting yourself – as worrying leads to inflammation in the body, which is also detrimental for health and wellbeing.

6. Maintain positive social connections

One of the yoga teachers conducted a small survey with her students, asking what they liked best about the yoga classes. While she might have expected to hear some positive feedback about the practices, the overwhelming response was about the valuable social aspects. Her students relish catching up with others and meeting for coffee after class. For some, especially those who live alone, the morning class is the only time they have social contact all day.

The communal side of yoga is also important for teachers. They have often taught the same students for many years, sometimes progressing to teaching grown-up children of their original students. So yoga creates community for students and teachers, both in a practical way (making new friends) and spiritual (feeling they belong) – facilitating positive connections and emotions that are essential to health and wellbeing.[67] In a culture that values individualism and where loneliness is common, especially in older age, the connection with others through yoga is a precious gift for students and teachers alike.[68] [69]

7. Find the right teacher and style of yoga to suit you

As the teachers here reiterated – when practising yoga, it is important to gain balance between under-using or over-exerting the body. Over the years, I have personally attended several yoga classes where the practice is like a gruelling gym workout with mega-strain and effort in attaining the poses. However, in my view, the aim of yoga is to fit the practice to the student not the student to the practice – anything else ignores unique individual anatomy. Not every student (or teacher) will be able to attain certain poses; for example, *Padmasana* (a challenging cross-legged, seated position where the feet are placed upon opposite thighs). Forcing feet and limbs into such positions risks severe injury. Better by far to work with compassion and allow the yoga practice to gently unfold as it helps to connect mind and body, and foster awareness of what each pose can teach within the limits of individual anatomy. If I received a dollar every time someone told me they are not flexible enough to do yoga I would be a very wealthy woman! The suppleness of both body and mind comes gradually with ongoing yoga practice, not the other way around.

In Australia there is no mandated qualification to become a yoga teacher, so just about anyone can hang out a sign and call themselves a teacher. Therefore, think carefully about who you entrust to instruct your body and mind about yoga. It pays to check the teacher's qualifications to find out how many hours of study they completed and whether they are currently engaging in ongoing professional development and training. There are a number of different organisations (as mentioned previously in this book, and listed below) that train or register yoga teachers. Information is available online and most have a search function by location that lists teachers who are members of their organisations, and provides contact information and details about classes:

- Yoga Australia
- International Yoga Teachers Association of Australia
- Dru International
- BKS Iyengar Yoga Association of Australia
- Yoga Alliance

There are also different traditions of yoga to choose from, ranging from the more physically-oriented Iyengar style, to gentler forms such as Dru. The teachers in this book often experimented with different styles before they found the right type of yoga for them. As they attest, it is important not to give up after the first class – there is a teacher and style of yoga out there to suit you.

Practising yoga leads to a more mindful, accepting and joyful approach to life, and can help people make the most of their later years. *So live as though you have the power to change the way you age, because you do.*

GLOSSARY

ASANA
Physical yoga poses or postures.

ASHTANGA YOGA
The eight-limbed system of yoga as described by Patanjali. It is also the name of a dynamic and physically vigorous style of yoga as promoted by Pattabhi Jois in Mysore, India.

BIKRAM YOGA
A challenging physical form of yoga, practised in a heated room with 26 set poses.

CHAKRA
Sanskrit for 'wheel' – referring to the seven energy centres in the body, which run along the spine, from the base of the spine to the crown of the head.

CAT POSE (MARJARIASANA)
This pose starts from a hands-and-knees tabletop position. On the out-breath the core muscles are pulled in towards the spine as the back rounds and the crown releases gently toward the floor. On the in-breath this pose is often paired with cow pose (bitilasana), whereby the belly sinks toward the floor, creating an arch in the back as the head rises.

DHARMA
The teachings of the Buddha, or an individual's purpose and path in life.

DOWNWARD DOG (ADHOMUKHA SVANASANA)
An inverted pose whereby the body forms an inverted V-shape with the feet and hands pressing into the floor and the hips pushing up towards the sky.

(THE) EIGHT LIMBS OF YOGA
Yama (ethical disciplines), *Niyama* (rules of conduct), *Asana* (postures), *Pranayama* (restraint or expansion of the breath), *Pratyahara* (withdrawal of the senses), *Dharana* (concentration), *Dhyana* (meditation) and *Samadhi* (absorption).

ESOTERIC STUDY
The study of ageless wisdom, particularly as presented in the theosophical writings and teachings of Alice Bailey.

GURU
A teacher.

HATHA YOGA
Hatha is the basic style of yoga, which forms the foundation for most styles of yoga. It has become a generic term for yoga that includes physical poses. In contemporary times it is often used to describe slower-paced classes with no flow to them.

HEADSTAND (SALAMBA SARVANGASANA)

The headstand is an advanced, inverted yoga pose, which is practised by resting the head and forearms in a triangular formation on the yoga mat.

INTEGRAL YOGA

Integral yoga is a gentle form of yoga based on the teachings of Swami Satchidananda (1914-2002).

IYENGAR YOGA

A style of yoga created by BKS Iyengar, which focuses on precision, detail and alignment in poses. It uses props, including yoga blocks or straps, to increase accessibility, or to assist with modifying the poses.

KARMA

The law of cause and effect. From a yogic perspective all thoughts, words and actions create karma, and this affects what happens across different lifetimes.

LEGS UP THE WALL (VIPARITA KARANI)

A restorative yoga pose performed lying on the back with the sit-bones close to the wall. From there the legs are extended up the wall so the backs of the legs rest against the wall itself.

MANTRA

A word or phrase chanted, such as *Om*.

MEDITATION
There are many traditions of meditation but most include a focus on stilling the flow of thoughts in the mind and being present in the here and now. Meditation is usually practised in a seated position with the eyes closed, although some physical movements, poetry and music can also have meditative qualities.

MODIFICATIONS
Variations made to yoga poses to make them suitable for different body types and conditions, for instance, degree of flexibility, injuries, pregnancy or trauma.

PATANJALI
The sage who compiled the Yoga Sutras as a guide on 'how to live' in order to advance along a spiritual path towards enlightenment.

POWER YOGA
A vigorous, physically challenging and flowing style of yoga derived from Ashtanga Yoga.

PRANA
Life energy; the breath or life force.

PRANAYAMA
Yogic breathing exercises to clear physical and emotional obstacles within the body, to free up the breath and enhance the flow of prana.

RESTORATIVE YOGA
Practising *asana* using props such as blocks, straps and blankets to allow the body to rest in comfort so it can relax more deeply.

SAVASANA
Also commonly known as corpse pose or relaxation pose; it involves lying on the back, on the floor, and is usually practised for several minutes at the end of a yoga class. It is one of the most important parts of a yoga practice as it helps to assimilate any changes resulting from the practice and allows the nervous system to settle.

SELF REALISATION
In yogic terms used to denote identification with the spiritual self as contrasted with one's material being (mind/body). Unification of one's human potential with one's divine potential. Also, a psychological term referring to finding one's life purpose.

SHOULDER STAND
An inverted pose which starts from lying down on the back. The hips and legs are taken up overhead and off the floor.

SUN SALUTATIONS (SURYA NAMASKAR)
A popular sequence of *asanas* often used to warm up the body at the start of a yoga class.

SWAMI
A yogi who has been initiated into a devout or traditional spiritual yoga community.

TRANSCENDENTAL MEDITATION
A meditation technique from the teaching of Maharishi Mahesh Yogi; it uses mantra or sound to help transcend the mind.

VINYASA
Yoga movements linked with the breath; a series of poses are strung together in a short or longer flow.

YOGA
To yoke or bind – union of body, breath and mind.

YOGA BLOCK
A yoga block is a rectangular-shaped block made from wood or dense foam, used as a prop in yoga practice. The purpose is to assist in stabilising poses or making them more accessible to students with different abilities, body types and conditions.

YOGA BOLSTER
A yoga bolster is typically a long, thick pillow or cushion, cylindrical or rectangular in shape. It is used as a prop in *asana* practice and relaxation, for instance, to cushion and align the body.

YOGA MAT
A yoga mat is made specifically for practising yoga on. Mats prevent the hands and feet from slipping during *asana* practice and because of this property they are also commonly called 'sticky mats'.

YOGA NIDRA

A long, guided relaxation/meditation technique usually performed in corpse pose (lying down).

YOGA STRAP

A yoga strap is a long belt made of nylon or cotton, with a buckle and D-ring at one end so the belt can be made into a loop as needed to assist in certain poses.

YOGA THERAPY (OR REMEDIAL YOGA)

The application of yoga, which may include: *asana*, meditation, breathing, diet, and changes to lifestyle to assist people who have physical and psychological conditions.

YOGI

A committed yoga practitioner. Yogini is often used to refer to a female practitioner; whereas a yogi is traditionally male.

PHOTO CAPTIONS AND CREDITS

Chapter 1

Tania practising yoga on the beach at Seatoun. Photo from Stuff/ Dominion Post.

Chapter 2

Maggie practising yoga in her garden. Photo provided by Maggie Coombs from her private collection, taken by a family member.

Maggie teaching a yoga class at Greenwich Point, 1980. Photo provided by Maggie Coombs, from her private collection, taken by a family member.

Chapter 3

Vivian on her 90th birthday. Photo provided by Vivian Vieritz from her private collection, taken by a family member.

Vivian aged 27 doing a handstand over her son Larry. Photo provided by Vivian Vieritz from her private collection, taken by a family member.

Vivian in her favourite pose, the headstand. Photo provided by Vivian Vieritz from her private collection, taken by a family member.

Chapter 4
Anita in her garden. Photo provided by Anita Clara, and taken by her partner Peter Schroeder.

Chapter 5
Susan in seated wide angle pose (upavishta konasana). Photo by Wyatt Dooley.

Chapter 6
Bette Calman in a 'cat suit'. Photo provided by Susanne Calman from her private collection.

Yoga with Bette Calman and poodle (circa 1980s). Photo by South Australian Magazine (SAM).

'A Smile', handout from Bette Calman's yoga class, circa mid-1990s. Courtesy of Bette Calman.

Chapter 7
Sheila at Twisting Fish Yoga Studio. Photo originally published in Western Suburbs Weekly, Perth, '84-year old Claremont yoga teacher proves age no barrier to healthy mind and body', 18th November 2016.

Chapter 8
Liz Coon. Photo provided by Liz Coon from her private collection.
Norm Coon. Photo provided by Liz Coon from her private collection.

Chapter 9

Judy Morgan. Photo provided by Judy Morgan. Courtesy Star Newspapers.

Judy Morgan practising yoga in 1971. Photo provided by Judy Morgan from her personal collection.

ACKNOWLEDGEMENTS

Endless thanks and gratitude to all the women who feature in this book for generously sharing their time and stories, yoga classes, photos and memories, and answering my never-ending questions: Judy Morgan, Vivian Vieritz, Susan Grbic, Bette Calman, Maggie Coombs, Tania Dyett, Anita Clara, Sheila Hays and Liz Coon. Also, thanks to their family members who provided assistance with photos and many other tasks: Susanne Calman, Kim Dyett and Larry Vieritz. A warm thanks to all the yoga teachers who participated in the wider research project on yoga and ageing. Although all their stories couldn't be included in the book, each one contributed to the wider project. My heartfelt thanks to Louise Bennett (Chintanshuddi) whose skill and talent made a valuable contribution in clarifying and ordering the manuscript. To the members of the Marion Writers Group (who at the start mostly knew nothing about yoga) for providing valuable feedback on drafts, and raising questions of clarification and encouragement. To Natalie Fuller for suggesting Barb St John's quote at the start of the book. Gaylene Denford-Wood for introducing me to Seminaria form, the diamond shaped poems, which feature at the start of each chapter. Shannon Griffin yoga teacher extraordinaire (and my teacher), who has been practising yoga for over 30 years but is still too young to feature in this book. And to Graham Stucley and my children Emma and Shaun for their love and support.

NOTES

Introduction

[1] World Health Organisation (2016) *Discrimination and Negative Attitudes about Ageing are Bad for Your Health*, News Release, Geneva, http:/www.who.int/news-room/detail/29-09-2016-discrimination-and-negative-attitudes-about-ageing

[2] Ibid.

[3] Joseph F. Coughlin (2017) *The Longevity Economy: Unlocking the World's Fastest-Growing, Most Misunderstood Market*, Public Affairs, Hachette Book Group, New York.

[4] Sat Bir Singh Khalsa, Lorenzo Cohen, Timothy McCall & Shirley Telles (2016) *The Principles and Practice of Yoga in Health Care*, Handspring Publishing, Edinburgh.

Chapter One: Tania's Story – Keeping The Body In Good Health With Yoga

[5] Referring to Giovanni Paolo Maggini, the 17th century Italian string maker.

[6] Lilias Folan is a famous American yoga teacher who had a television program called *Lilias, Yoga and You*, which aired from the 1970s to the 1990s.

[7] Lilias Folan (1976) *Yoga and You*, Bantam Books, New York.

[8] Geshe Tashi Tsering (2005) *Four Noble Truths: The Foundations of Buddhist Thought*, Volume 1, Wisdom Books, Somerville, MA, p.24.

Chapter Two: Maggie's Story – Yoga Is The Best Option

[9] Michael Volin opened one of the first yoga schools in Sydney, in the mid-1950s.

[10] Arriving in Australia from India in 1967, Swami Sarasvati became Australia's foremost yoga expert when she presented a regular yoga program on commercial television.

[11] Nancy Phelan was a prominent Australian writer who published several books on yoga.

[12] Russell Frank Atkinson (1990) *Diary of a Dropout*, Wellspring, Mosman Junction, NSW.

[13] Born in a village in Assam (India), Acharya lived a traditional rural life as a child and developed an interest in spirituality at a young age.

[14] Swamiji Kamala-Mata Aranya was English born and came to Australia to set up the Aranya Ashram in the Atherton Tablelands (Queensland).

Chapter Three: Vivian's Story – You're Never Too Old To Practise Yoga

[15] BKS Iyengar was the founder of the style of modern yoga known as 'Iyengar Yoga' and was considered one of the foremost yoga teachers in the world. He also authored many books on yoga practice and philosophy.

[16] Tammy Williams has been running yoga teacher training, mindfulness training, yoga retreats and events across Australia for many years.

Chapter Four: Anita's Story – Changing From The Inside-Out

[17] Ian Gawler was a pioneer in Australia in popularising meditation. He used meditation and dietary changes in his own fight against bone cancer, which was declared cured in 1978 (Guy Allenby (2008) Ian Gawler, *The Dragon's Blessing*, Allen and Unwin, Crows Nest, NSW).

[18] The Eight Limbs of yoga are: *Yama* (ethical disciplines), *Niyama* (rules of conduct), *Asana* (postures), *Pranayama* (restraint or expansion of the breath), *Pratyahara* (withdrawal of the senses), *Dharana* (concentration), *Dhyana* (meditation) and *Samadhi* (absorption).

[19] Dru Yoga is a style of yoga that has its foundations set in ancient yogic tradition, and includes soft flowing movements, directed breathing and visualisation.

[20] Chris Barrington is one of the founders of Dru Yoga.

[21] Erich Schiffmann (1996) *Yoga, The Spirit and Practice of Moving into Stillness*, Pocket Books, New York, p.4.

Chapter Five: Susan's Story – Growing Younger Through Yoga

[22] TM refers to a specific form of silent mantra meditation. Maharishi Mahesh Yogi created and introduced the TM technique and spiritual movement in India in the mid-1950s.

[23] Sant Mat translates as the Teachings of the Saints: a universal, non-denominational spiritual path.

[24] Iyengar Yoga (developed by BKS Iyengar) is a form of Hatha

Yoga with emphasis on precision and alignment in posture (*asana*) and breath control (*pranayama*).

[25] Integral Yoga synthesizes classical yoga philosophy and practice, including: Hatha, Raja, Bhakti, Karma, Jnana, and Japa Yoga. It was brought to the West from India by Swami Satchidananda Saraswati.

[26] Referring to where a teacher touches the student to correct a pose, as well as to aid awareness.

[27] Donna Farhi is a renowned yoga teacher whose wisdom and expertise are keenly sought after. Based in rural north Canterbury near Christchurch (New Zealand) she has 39 years of experience in teaching yoga.

[28] Ashtanga Yoga was created by K Pattabhi Jois during the 20th century, and often promoted as a modern-day form of classical Indian yoga.

[29] Bikram Yoga became popular in the early 1970s and is a system of yoga that Bikram Choudhury synthesized from traditional Hatha Yoga techniques.

[30] Ellen Langer (2009) *Counterclockwise: Mindful Health and the Power of Possibility*, Hodder & Stoughton, London, p.11.

[31] Joseph F. Coughlin (2017) *The Longevity Economy, Unlocking the World's Fastest-Growing, Most Misunderstood Market*, Public Affairs, Hachette Book Group, New York.

Chapter Six: Bette's Story – Relax, Reset And Recharge The Body

[32] Nancy Phelan and Michael Volin (1963) *Yoga for Women*, Harper, New York.

[33] Dukes was a fascinating man. Aside from a passion for yoga, he worked for the British Secret Intelligence Service and was renowned as a master of disguises. In 1920, he was knighted for his exploits in espionage by King George V.

[34] Selvarajan Yesudian and Elisabeth Haich (1953) *Yoga and Health,* Harper Brothers, New York.

Yesudian and Haich founded the first yoga school in Budapest, but it closed when the communist regime took over after the Second World War. Afterwards they established a yoga school in Switzerland, which became one of the largest and oldest yoga schools in Europe.

[35] Michael Volin was born in Russia and lived in China for a while before moving to Australia in the late 1940s.

[36] Iris Clutterham founded the Yoga Teachers Institute of South Australia (YTISA) in 1950.

[37] Bette Calman and Joan Brodie (1977) *Yoga for Arthritis*, Rigby Instant Book, Rigby, Adelaide; Bette Calman and Joan Brodie (1975) *Yoga for Weight Control*, Rigby Instant Book, Rigby, Adelaide; Bette Calman and Joan Brodie (1977) *Yoga for Relaxation*, Rigby Instant Book, Rigby, Adelaide.

Chapter Seven: Sheila's Story – Safe Yoga For Seniors

[38] The Rishikesh sequence was introduced to the west by Swami Sivananda, and is named after the Rishikesh region at the foot of the Himalayas (where it originated). The sequence forms part of the Sivananda Yoga tradition.

[39] The first series about yoga on British TV was with Sir Paul Dukes, on the BBC in 1951, which comprised a series of four programs.

[40] The idea of *Flower Power* originated in Berkley, California as a symbol of protesting against the Vietnam War. It involved passive resistance and non-violence using flowers as a symbol of peace and love.

[41] Wilfred Clark encouraged the growth of yoga in Birmingham in the 1960s, and set up the Wheel of British Yoga in 1965, which was the forerunner to the British Wheel of Yoga. He wanted to broaden interest in yoga to different regions across Britain.

[42] The Eight Limbs of yoga are: *Yama* (ethical disciplines), *Niyama* (rules of conduct), *Asana* (postures), *Pranayama* (restraint or expansion of the breath), *Pratyahara* (withdrawal of the senses), *Dharana* (concentration), *Dhyana* (meditation) and *Samadhi* (absorption).

Chapter Eight: Liz's Story – A Yearning To Exercise

[43] Woodhouse, Fay (2014) 'So new and exotic! Gita Yoga in Australia from the 1950s to today' (online article) *Victorian Historical Journal*, Vol. 85, No. 2, Dec, pp. 299–320. Availability: https://search.informit.com.au/documentSummary; dn=928602571763859;res=IELAPA> ISSN: 1030-7710. [Cited 11 Sep 18].

[44] Bikram Yoga is adapted from traditional yoga by Bikram Choudhury. It is a 'hot yoga' style, generally practised in a room heated to specific temperatures.

[45] Commonly referred to as *'flow yoga'*, *Vinyasa* is a style of yoga born from the *Ashtanga* lineage and modernised by Patthabi Jois.

[46] Iyengar Yoga is a form of Hatha Yoga that has an emphasis on detail, precision and alignment in the performance of posture

(*asana*) and breath control (*pranayama*). Strength, mobility and stability are gained through the *asanas*. Mr Iyengar visited Australia in 1983 and 1992.

[47] BKS Iyengar (1966) *Light on Yoga*, George Allen and Unwin, Great Britain.

[48] Ashtanga Vinyasa Yoga was founded by K Pattabhi Jois during the 20th century, and is a style of classical India yoga adapted for the modern world. Ashtanga focuses on a flowing sequence of postures.

Chapter Nine: Judy's Story – Giving The Gift Of Yoga

[49] Michael Volin opened the Sydney Yoga Centre in 1950. His classes were extremely popular and he went on to author several books on yoga.

[50] The *Pawanmuktasana Series One* is a simple, gentle preparatory set of practices that exercise all the major joints of the body and relax the muscles. It is suitable where vigorous physical exercise isn't advisable. From *Asana Pranayama Mudra Bandha*, Swami Satyananda Saraswati (2008) Yoga Publications Trust, Munger, Bihar, India.

[51] From David S. Viscott (1993) *Finding Your Strength in Difficult Times: A Book of Meditations*, Contemporary Books of Chicago, Illinois, p.87.

Chapter Ten: Practise Yoga For Radiant Ageing

[52] Marcy C. McCall (2013) How Might Yoga Work? An Overview of Potential Underlying Mechanisms, Research Article, *Journal of Yoga and Physical Therapy,* 3(1), pp. 1–7.

[53] Roderik J. S. Gerritsen and Guido P. H. Band (2018) Breath of Life: The Respiratory Vagal Stimulation Model of Contemplative Activity, *Frontiers in Human Neuroscience*, Vol. 12, p. 397. Yogic breathing (diaphragmatic breathing) is thought to stimulate the vagus nerve, which forms part of the calming parasympathetic nervous system.

[54] Marcy C. McCall (2013) How Might Yoga Work? op. cit.

[55] Denise Taylor (2012) Review: Physical Activity is Medicine for Older Adults, *BMJ*, 90, p. 1059.

[56] Alice Tulloch, Hannah Bombell, Catherine Dean and Anne Tiedemann (2018) Yoga-based Exercise Improves Health-related Quality of Life and Mental Well-being in Older people: A Systematic Review of Randomised Controlled Trials, *Age and Ageing,* Vol. 47(4), July 2018, pp. 537–544.

[57] Leonardo Barbosa Barreto de Brito, Djalma Rabelo Ricardo and Denise Sardinha Mendes Soares de Araújo (2012) Ability to Sit and Rise from the Floor as a Predictor of All-cause Mortality, *European Journal of Preventative Cardiology,* Vol. 21(7), pp. 892–898. Musculoskeletal fitness was assessed by a sitting rising test (SRT) with 2,002 adults (aged 51-80). Lower SRT tests scores were a predictor of all-cause mortality.

[58] John Darwin (2014) Mindful Aging: Become a Hero, Centre for Mindful Life Enhancement Discussion Paper https://www.mindfulenhance.org/other-resources/discussion-papers

[59] Alyson Ross, Margaret Bevans, Erika Friedmann, Laurie Williams and Sue Thomas (2014) "I Am a Nice Person When I Do Yoga!!!" A Qualitative Analysis of How Yoga Affects Relationships, *Journal of Holistic Nursing*, 32(2), pp. 67–77.

[60] Mihaly Csikszentmihalyi (2013) *Flow: The Classic Work on How to Achieve Happiness*, Random House, London.

[61] Barbara Humberstone and Carol Cutler-Riddick (2015) Older Women, Embodiment and Yoga Practice, *Ageing and Society*, Vol. 35(6), pp. 1221–1241.

[62] D.L. Katz and S. Meller (2014) Can We Say What Diet Is Best for Health? *Annual Review of Public Health*, 35, pp. 83–103. Gene expression is the process whereby the information contained in a gene becomes a useful product.

[63] Ibid.

[64] Mariette Gerber and Richard Hoffman (2015) The Mediterranean Diet: Health, Science and Society, *British Journal of Nutrition*, 113, Suppl 2: S4-10. The authors found some evidence for the benefits of a Mediterranean diet, but in its entirety with olive oil, moderate meat consumption and meat consumption of raised non-intensive farming in conjunction with a lifestyle of physical activity.

[65] D.L. Katz and S. Meller (2014) op. cit.

[66] Yoga has a philosophy of non-violence or non-harming (ahimsa) to others. This can be interpreted in different ways, including as not to harm animals by choosing to be vegetarian. For individuals with particular medical conditions or dietary needs, eating meat may equate to practising non-violence or non-harming towards their own bodies.

[67] Alyson Ross, Margaret Bevans, Erika Friedmann, Laurie Williams and Sue Thomas (2014) op. cit.

[68] Many study findings (including the following) show the negative effects of loneliness and isolation on health and wellbeing: Holwerda T.J., van Tilburg T.G., Deeg D.J.H., Schutter N., Dekker J., Stek M.L., Beekman A.T.F., Schoevers R.A. and Rien V. (2016) Impact of Loneliness and Depression on Mortality: Results from the Longitudinal Ageing Study Amsterdam, *Br. J. Psychiatry*, 209, pp. 127–134; Valtorta N.K., Kanaan M., Gilbody S., Ronzi S. and Hanratty B. (2016) Loneliness and Social Isolation as Risk Factors for Coronary Heart Disease and Stroke: Systematic Review and Meta-analysis of Longitudinal Observational Studies, *Heart,* 102, pp. 1009–1016.

[69] Barbara Humberstone and Carol Cutler-Riddick (2015) op. cit.

ABOUT THE AUTHOR

Associate Professor Kathy Arthurson is an internationally recognised social scientist, writer and researcher. She also teaches mindfulness and life skills to university students (Flinders University). For over twenty years, she has practised and taught yoga (kathyarthursonyoga.com). She lives with her partner in Adelaide (South Australia) – recently voted the world's tenth most liveable city.